Health Care Policy

READINGS IN BIOETHICS

Edited by Thomas A. Shannon

Readings in Bioethics is a series of anthologies that gather together seminal essays in four areas: reproductive technologies, genetic technologies, death and dying, and health care policy. Each of the readers addresses specific case studies and issues under its respective topic. The goal of this series is twofold: first, to provide a set of readers on thematic topics for introductory or survey courses in bioethics or for courses with a particular theme or time limitation. When used in conjunction with a core text that provides the appropriate level of analytical framework, the readers in this series provide specific analysis of a set of issues that meets the professor's individual needs and interests. Second, each of the readers in this series is designed with the student in mind and aims to present seminal articles and case studies that help students focus more thoroughly and effectively on specific topics that flesh out the ethical issues at the core of bioethics.

Volumes in the Readings in Bioethics Series:

Reproductive Technologies
Genetic Technologies
Death and Dying
Health Care Policy

Health Care Policy

A Reader

Edited by
Thomas A. Shannon

A SHEED & WARD BOOK

ROWMAN & LITTLEFIELD PUBLISHERS, INC.
Lanham • Boulder • New York • Toronto • Oxford

A SHEED & WARD BOOK

ROWMAN & LITTLEFIELD PUBLISHERS, INC.

Published in the United States of America
by Rowman & Littlefield Publishers, Inc.
A wholly owned subsidiary of The Rowman & Littlefield Publishing Group, Inc.
4501 Forbes Boulevard, Suite 200, Lanham, Maryland 20706
www.rowmanlittlefield.com

PO Box 317
Oxford
OX2 9RU, UK

British Library Cataloguing in Publication Information Available

Library of Congress Cataloging-in-Publication Data

Health care policy : a reader / edited by Thomas A. Shannon.
    p. cm.
    "A Sheed & Ward Book"
    Includes bibliographical references and index.
    ISBN 0-7425-3215-1 (cloth : alk. paper) —ISBN 0-7425-3216-X (pbk. : alk. paper)
    1. Medical policy. 2. Medical policy—Moral and ethical aspects. 3. Bioethics.
I. Shannon, Thomas A. (Thomas Anthony), 1940–
RA395.A3H41245 2004
362.1—dc22

                                                                    2004005729

Printed in the United States of America

⊗™ The paper used in this publication meets the minimum requirements of American
National Standard for Information Sciences—Permanence of Paper for Printed Library
Materials, ANSI/NISO Z39.48-1992.

To my colleagues and friends

James Keenan, SJ
Thomas J. Massaro, SJ
Ed Vacek, SJ
Ken Himes, OFM
James J. Walter

With gratitude for
your many acts of generosity and support

Contents

Acknowledgments

Gratefully acknowledged are the publishers and authors of the works listed below for their permission to reprint their publications.

Norman Daniels. "Justice, Health, and Healthcare." *American Journal of Bioethics* 1 (Spring 2001): 2-16. Reprinted by permission of the author.

Kevin M. De Cock and Robert S. Janssen, "An Unequal Epidemic in an Unequal World." *Journal of the American Medical Association* 288 (10 July 2002): 236-238. Reprinted by permission of the American Medical Association.

Esteban González Burchard, Elad Ziv, Natasha Coyle, Scarlett Lin Gomez, Hua Tang, Andrew J. Karter, Joanna L. Mountain, Eliseo J. Pérez-Stable, Dean Sheppard, and Neil Risch. "The Importance of Race and Ethnic Background in Biomedical Research and Clinical Practice." *New England Journal of Medicine* 348 (20 March 2003): 1170-1175. Copyright © 2003. Reprinted by permission of the Massachusetts Medical Society. All rights reserved.

Lawrence O. Gostin, Jason W. Sapsin, Stephen P. Teret, Scott Burris, Julie Samia Mair, James G. Hodge, Jr., and Jon S. Vernick. "The Model State Emergency Health Powers Act." *Journal of the American Medical Association* 288 (7 August 2002): 622-628. Reprinted by permission of the American Medical Association.

Hamilton Moses III, Eugene Braunwald, Joseph B. Martin, and Samuel O. Their. "Collaborating with Industry—Choices for the Academic Medical Center." *New England Journal of Medicine* 347 (24 October 2002): 1371-1375. Copyright © 2002. Reprinted by permission of the Massachusetts Medical Society. All rights reserved.

Scott D. Halpern, Jason H. T. Karlawish, and Jesse A. Berlin. "The Continuing Unethical Conduct of Underpowered Clinical Trials." *Journal of the American Medical Association* 288 (17 July 2002): 358-362. Reprinted by permission of the American Medical Association.

Diane M. Reddy, Raymond Fleming, and Carolyne Swain. "Effect of Mandatory Parental Notification on Adolescent Girls' Use of Sexual Health Care Services."

Journal of the American Medical Association 288 (14 August 2002): 710-714.
Reprinted by permission of the American Medical Association.
Madhav Goyal, Ravindra L. Mehta, Lawrence J. Schneiderman, and Ashwini R.
Sehgal. "Economic and Health Consequences of Selling a Kidney in India." *Journal of the American Medical Association* 288 (2 October 2002): 1589-1593.
Reprinted by permission of the American Medical Association.
Peter Monaghan. "Scholarly Watchdogs for an Ethical Netherworld." *The Chronicle of Higher Education* (6 October 2000). A3-A4. Copyright 2000. Reprinted by permission of *The Chronicle of Higher Education*.
Susan L. Mitchell, Joan M. Teno, Jason Roy, Glen Kabumoto, Vincent Mor. "Clinical and Organizational Factors Associated with Feeding Tube Use among Nursing Home Residents with Advanced Cognitive Impairment." *Journal of the American Medical Association* 290 (2 July 2003): 73-80. Reprinted by permission of the American Medical Association.
Robin A. Weiss, "Xenografts and Retroviruses." *Science* 285 (20 August 1999): 1221-1222. Copyright © 1999 AAAS. Reprinted by permission of *Science* Magazine.
Ethics Committee of the American Society for Reproductive Medicine. "Donating Spare Embryos for Embryonic Stem-Cell Research." *Fertility and Sterility* 78 (November 2002): 957-960. Copyright © 2002. Reprinted by permission of The American Society of Reproductive Medicine.

Introduction

Since its introduction over a decade ago, the field of bioethics has grown exponentially. Not only has it become established as an academic discipline with journals and professional societies, it is covered regularly in the media and affects people everyday around the globe.

One important development in the field has been the informal division into clinical and institutional bioethics. Institutional bioethics has to do with the ethical dilemmas associated with the various institutions, the majority of which are providers of health care services. Delivery of health care, allocations of health care payments, mergers, closing or restricting services of certain departments or even of hospitals or clinics themselves are systemic questions involving a broad range of ethical agenda. On the clinical side, the bevy of usual suspects of ethical dilemmas is increasing in complexity as technology moves forward, new interventions are proposed, and fantasies become realities. Few, for example, thought that human cloning would become a serious clinical, public policy, and institutional debate in 2002.

One of the major consequences of this quantitative and qualitative debate is that providing resources for introductory or even specialized courses is becoming much more difficult. This is particularly difficult in the case of editing an anthology to complement a text that provides an analysis of the core ethical issues. There is simply too much material to put into a single anthology that is reasonable in price and convenient in size.

This series is an attempt to resolve the problem of a cumbersome and expensive anthology by providing a set of four manageable and accessible readers on specific topics. Thus each reader in the series will be on a specific topic—reproductive technologies, genetic technologies, death and dying, and health care policy—and will be about two hundred pages in length. This is to provide professors with flexibility in designing their courses. Ideally, professors will use a core text to analyze the primary ethical issues in bioethics and will use the readers in this series to examine specific problems and cases, thus providing flexibility in designing syllabi as well as providing variety in presenting the course.

The goal of this series is twofold: first, to provide a set of readers on thematic topics for introductory or survey courses in bioethics or for courses with a particular theme or time limitation. In addition to a core text that provides the appropriate level of analytical framework, the readers in this series provide specific analysis of a set of issues that meets the professor's needs and interests. Second, each of the readers in this series is designed with the student in mind and aims to present seminal articles and case studies that help students focus more thoroughly and effectively on specific topics that flesh out the ethical issues at the core of bioethics.

1

Justice, Health, and Healthcare

Norman Daniels

Healthcare (including public health) is special because it protects normal functioning, which in turn protects the range of opportunities open to individuals. I extend this account in two ways. First, since the distribution of goods other than healthcare affect population health and its distribution, I claim that Rawls's principles of justice describe a fair distribution of the social determinants of health, giving a partial account of when health inequalities are unjust. Second, I supplement a principled account of justice for health and healthcare with an account of fair process for setting limits or rationing care. This account is provided by three conditions that comprise "accountability for reasonableness."

THREE QUESTIONS OF JUSTICE

A theory of justice for health and healthcare should help us answer three central questions. First, is healthcare special? Is it morally important in ways that justify (and explain) the fact that many societies distribute healthcare more equally than many other social goods? Second, when are health inequalities unjust? After all, many socially controllable factors besides access to healthcare affect the levels of population health and the degree of health inequalities in a population. Third, how can we meet competing healthcare needs fairly under reasonable resource constraints? General principles of justice that answer the first two questions do not, I argue, answer some important questions about rationing fairly. Is there instead a fair process for making rationing decisions?

1

About twenty years ago I answered the first question by claiming health-care was special because of its impact on opportunity (Daniels 1981, 1985). Specifically, the central function of healthcare is to maintain normal functioning. Disease and disability, by impairing normal functioning, restrict the range of opportunities open to individuals. Healthcare thus makes a distinct but limited contribution to the protection of equality of opportunity. Though I construed healthcare broadly to include public health as well as individual preventive, acute, and chronic care, I ignored other factors that have a profound effect on population health. Unfortunately, focusing on just healthcare adds to the popular misconception that our vastly improved health in the last century is primarily the result of healthcare.

During the last twenty years, a major literature has emerged exploring the social determinants of health. We have long known that the richer people are, the longer and healthier their lives. The powerful findings of the last couple of decades, however, have deepened our understanding of the factors at work producing these effects on population health and the distribution of health within populations. It is less tenable to think that it is simply poverty and true deprivation that diminishes the health of some people, for there is growing evidence that race and class effects operate across a broad range of inequalities. Since social policies—not laws of human nature or economic development—are responsible for the social and economic inequalities that produce these health effects, we are forced to look upstream from the point of medical delivery and ask about the fairness of the distribution of these goods. Rawls's theory of justice as fairness, quite serendipitously, contains principles that give a plausible account of the fair distribution of those determinants, thus providing an answer to the second question (Daniels, Kennedy, and Kawachi 1999, 2000).

During the 1980s I became aware that my account of just healthcare, like other general theories, failed to give specific guidance, or gave implausible answers, to certain questions about rationing (Daniels 1993). Though philosophers may work out middle-level principles that can supplement general accounts of distributive justice and solve these unsolved rationing problems, it is unlikely that there will be consensus on them in the foreseeable future. Distributive issues remain highly contested.

In the absence of consensus on distribution principles, we need a fair process to establish legitimacy for critical resource allocation decisions. My account of a fair process for addressing these distributive issues is called "accountability for reasonableness" (Daniels and Sabin 1997, 1998a, n.d.). It is an attempt to connect views about deliberative democracy to decision making at various institutional levels, whether public or private, in our complex health systems.

My goal in this essay is to sketch the central ideas behind my approach to all three questions and to suggest how they all fit together. Detailed arguments can be found in the references. By pursing a theory of justice toward providing answers to all three questions, and not simply the first, I hope to give a fuller demonstration that justice is good for our health.

WHAT IS THE SPECIAL MORAL IMPORTANCE OF HEALTHCARE?

The central moral importance, for purposes of justice, of preventing and treating disease and disability with effective healthcare services (construed broadly to include public health and environmental measures, as well as personal medical services) derives from the way in which protecting normal functioning contributes to protecting opportunity.[1] Specifically, by keeping people close to normal functioning, healthcare preserves for people the ability to participate in the political, social, and economic life of their society. It sustains them as fully participating citizens—normal collaborators and competitors—in all spheres of social life.

By maintaining normal functioning, healthcare protects an individual's fair share of the normal range of opportunities (or plans of life) reasonable people would choose in a given society. This normal opportunity range is societally relative, dependent on various facts about the society's level of technological development and social organization. Individuals' fair shares of that societal normal opportunity range are the plans of life it would be reasonable for them to choose were they not ill or disabled and were their talents and skills suitably protected against mis- or underdevelopment as a result of unfair social practices and the consequences of socioeconomic inequalities. Individuals generally choose to develop only some of their talents and skills, effectively narrowing their range of opportunities. Maintaining normal functioning preserves, however, their broader, fair share of the normal opportunity range, giving them the chance to revise their plans of life over time.

This relationship between healthcare and the protection of opportunity suggests that the appropriate principle of distributive justice for regulating the design of a healthcare system is a principle protecting equality of opportunity. Any theory of justice that supports a principle assuring equal opportunity (or giving priority to improving the opportunities of those who have the least opportunity) could thus be extended to healthcare. At the time I proposed this approach, the best defense of such a general principle was to be found in Rawls's theory of justice as fairness (Rawls 1971). One of the principles Rawls's social contractors would choose is a principle assuring them *fair equality of opportunity* in access to jobs and offices. This principle not only prohibits discriminatory barriers to access, but requires positive social measures that correct for the negative effects on opportunity, including the underdevelopment of skills and talents, that derive from unfair social practices (e.g., a legacy of gender or race bias) or socioeconomic inequalities. Such positive measures would include among other things the provision of public education and other opportunity-improving early childhood interventions.

Rawls, however, had deliberately simplified the formulation of his general theory of justice by assuming that people are fully functional over a normal life span. His social contractors thus represented people who suffered no disease or disability or premature death. By subsuming the protection of normal functioning under (a suitably adjusted version of) his principle assuring fair equality of opportunity, I showed how to drop that idealization and apply his theory to the real world. (Rawls (1993) supports this approach.) In the last two decades, however, other work on egalitarianism has suggested alternative ways to connect healthcare to opportunity or to positive liberty or capabilities, and I shall comment on them shortly. First, I want to highlight some key elements of my approach.

The fair equality of opportunity account does not use the impact of disease or disability on welfare (desire satisfaction, happiness, or utility) or utility as a basis for thinking about distributive justice. One might have thought, for example, that what was special about healthcare was that good health was important for happiness. But illness and disability may not lead to unhappiness, even if they restrict the range of opportunities open to an individual. Intuitively, then, there is something attractive about locating the moral importance of meeting healthcare needs in the more objective impact on opportunity than in the more subjective impact on happiness.

This analysis fits well with and extends Rawls's (1971) nonwelfarist account of primary social goods. For purposes of justice, Rawls argued, we should not seek to determine what we owe each other by measuring our satisfaction or welfare, but we should measure our levels of well-being by publicly accessible measures. For Rawls this means an index of primary social goods that includes rights and liberties, power and opportunity, income and wealth, and the social bases of self-respect. My account includes the protection of normal functioning within the scope of the primary good of opportunity. Drawing on insights from Scanlon's (1975) discussion of the "urgency" of meeting some "preferences" to relieve decrements in well-being but not others, my account explains why we believe we have obligations to assist others in meeting healthcare needs but not necessarily to provide them with other things they say they need to make them happier.

Consider an actual issue where the contrast is important. People with longstanding disabilities will often rank their welfare higher than do people who are merely imagining life with such disabilities. Perhaps people with disabilities accommodate by adjusting their goals and expectations. Even if they are more satisfied with their lives than people without disabilities might expect, there is an objective loss in their range of capabilities and opportunities, and that loss is captured by the appeal to a fair share of an opportunity range. The fair equality of opportunity account thus avoids a troubling feature that haunts cost-utility analysis and its treatment of such disabilities.[2]

Healthcare is of special moral importance because it helps to preserve our status as fully functioning citizens. By itself, however, this does not distinguish healthcare from food, shelter, and rest, which also meet basic needs of citizens by preserving normal functioning. Since medical needs are more unequally distributed than these other needs and can be catastrophically expensive, they are appropriately seen as the object of private or social insurance schemes. It might be argued that we can finesse the problem of talking about the medical needs we feel we are obliged to meet for one another if we assure people fair income shares from which they can purchase such insurance. We cannot, however, define a minimal but fair income share unless it is capable of meeting such needs (Daniels 1985).

Some economists and philosophers may object that giving special status to health insurance will be "paternalistic" and inefficient since some people prefer to trade income for things other than healthcare.[3] Our social obligation, however, is to provide institutions (such as social insurance or subsidies to buy private insurance) that protect opportunity, not to maximize aggregate welfare or achieve efficiency above all else. The principles of justice defended here thus depart from utilitarian goals.

The account sketched here has several implications for the design of our healthcare institutions and for issues of resource allocation. Perhaps most important, the account supports the provision of universal access to appropriate healthcare—including traditional public health and preventive measures—through public or mixed public and private insurance schemes. Healthcare aimed at protecting fair equality of opportunity should not be distributed according to ability to pay, and the burden of payment should not fall disproportionately on the ill (Daniels 1985, 1995; and Daniels, Light, and Caplan 1996).

Properly designed universal coverage health systems will be constrained by reasonable budgets, since healthcare is not the only important good. Reasonable resource constraints will then require judgments about which medical needs are more important to meet than others. Priority setting and rationing is thus a requirement of justice, since meeting healthcare needs should not and need not be a bottomless pit.

The elderly might object that an opportunity based account of just healthcare will leave them out in the cold, for their opportunities might seem to be in the past. We can avoid this by not biasing our allocations in favor of one stage of life and instead considering the age-relative opportunity range. Still, treating people differently at different stages of life—for example, saving resources from one stage of life for use at another—does not produce inequalities across persons in the way that differential treatment by race or gender does. We all age—though we do not change gender or race. Fairness between age groups in designing a healthcare system is appropriately modeled by the idea of prudent allocation over a life span (Daniels 1988). Under some conditions of scarcity, this implies that "pure" rationing by age (where age is not proxy for other traits) is permissible.[4]

Some universal coverage healthcare systems permit a supplementary tier that is purchased by those who are best off in society. For example, the British private insurance sector allows about 10% of the population to have quicker access to services that others must wait longer for in the British National Health Service. Other countries, such as Norway, prohibit a supplementary tier, fearing it will undermine the political solidarity needed to sustain their generous healthcare system. The fair equality of opportunity account constrains, but does not rule out, all tiering (Daniels 1998a; Daniels, Light, and Caplan 1996).

One controversial implication of my approach provides a way to contrast the fair equality of opportunity view with some alternative egalitarian accounts. In aiming at normal functioning, my approach views the prevention and treatment of disease and disability as the primary rationale for what we owe each other by way of assistance in co-operative healthcare schemes (Buchanan et al. 2000). Enhancing otherwise normal conditions—even when they put us at a disadvantage compared to others through no fault of our own—is then viewed as "not medically necessary." For example, there is support in my view for the common insurance practice of covering treatment for very short children who have growth hormone deficiencies but not covering it for equally short children who are otherwise normal.

The objection to my view is that this coverage policy seems to place too much weight on the presence of disease and disability and too little on what really should matter to an account aiming at protecting opportunity, namely, reducing the disadvantage that extreme shortness brings. This objection might be pressed by those who defend "equal opportunity for welfare or advantage" (Arneson 1988; G. A. Cohen 1989). Their view rests on the claim that anyone who suffers bad "brute luck"—a deficit in welfare or advantage that is no fault of their own—has a claim on others for assistance or compensation. In contrast, bad "option luck," the result of the choices we make or are responsible for making, does not give rise to claims on others. A disadvantage in talents or skills or even height that is not our fault thus provides a basis for claims on others for compensation or possibly enhancement. I argue (Daniels

1990, 2000a) that this view gives too much centrality to choice or responsibility, a centrality we do not and should not recognize when we want to protect our capabilities as citizens in a democratic society; there are good policy objections to this view as well (Sabin and Daniels 1994).

A similar objection might be raised from a perspective grounded in the importance of positive liberty or freedom, thought of as our capability to do or be what we choose (Sen 1980, 1992, 1999). The claim is that we should not necessarily be focused on a concept such as disease or disability but rather on whether individuals have the appropriate set of capabilities to do or be what they choose. Perhaps the very short child who is otherwise normal still lacks a key trait or capability that we should address.

If we consider more carefully, however, when differences in capabilities give rise to claims on others, support for treating the short but normal child may disappear. Sen (1992) himself notes that many differences in capabilities will be "incommensurable," since there will be no consensus about whether a person is worse off than others. The short but normal child, for example, may have an excellent temperament or wonderful social or cognitive skills. The cases where there is likely to be agreement that someone is clearly worse off in capabilities are likely to be captured by the categories of (serious) disease and disability. In practice, then, this view converges much more with the view I defend than it may appear at first.[5]

These alternative views obviously deserve more careful discussion than I can offer here. Still, my answer to the original question, that the special moral importance of healthcare derives from the protection of our opportunities, remains a defensible member of a family of views connecting healthcare to our opportunities and capabilities. Moreover, its practical implications converge more with those of its cousins than is apparent from the family quarrels among them.

WHICH HEALTH INEQUALITIES ARE UNJUST?

Universal access to appropriate healthcare—just healthcare—does not break the link between social status and health that I noted earlier, a point driven home in studies of the effects on health inequality of the British National Health Service (Black et al. 1988; Acheson et al. 1998; Marmot et al. 1998), and confirmed by work in other countries as well (Kawachi, Kennedy, and Wilkinson 1999). Our health is affected not simply by the ease with which we can see a doctor—though that surely matters—but also by our social position and the underlying inequality of our society. We cannot, of course, infer causation from these correlations between social inequality and health inequality (though later I explore some ideas about how the one might lead to the other). Suffice to say that, while the exact processes are not fully understood, the evidence suggests that there are social determinants of health (Marmot 1999).

If social factors play a large role in determining our health, then efforts to ensure greater justice in health outcomes should not focus simply on the traditional health sector. Health is produced not merely by having access to medical prevention and treatment, but also—to a measurably greater extent—by the cumulative experience of social conditions over the course of one's life. By the time a sixty-year-old heart attack victim arrives at the emergency room, bodily insults have accumulated over a lifetime. For such a person, medical care is, figuratively speaking, "the ambulance waiting at the bottom of the cliff." Much contemporary discussion about reducing health inequalities by increasing access to medical care misses this point. Of course, we still want that ambulance there, but we should be looking as well to improve social conditions that help to determine the health of societies.

As I noted earlier, Rawls's theory of justice as fairness was not designed to address issues of healthcare. He assumed a completely healthy population, and argued that a just society must assure people equal basic liberties, guarantee that the right of political participation has roughly equal value for all, provide a robust form of equal opportunity, and limit inequalities to those that benefit the least advantaged. When these requirements of justice are met, Rawls argued, we can have reasonable confidence that others are showing us the respect that is essential to our sense of self-worth. The fair terms of cooperation specified by these principles promote our social and political well-being.

The conjecture I explore is that by establishing equal liberties, robustly equal opportunity, a fair distribution of resources, and support for our self-respect—the basics of Rawlsian justice—we would go a long way toward eliminating the most important injustices in health outcomes. To be sure, social justice is valuable for reasons other than its effects on health (or Rawls could not have set aside issues of health when arguing for justice as fairness). And social reform in the direction of greater justice would not eliminate the need to think hard about fair allocation of resources within the healthcare system. Still, acting to promote social justice is a crucial step toward improving our health because there is this surprising convergence between what is needed for our social and political well-being and for our mental and physical health.

To see the basis for this conjecture about Rawlsian principles, let us review very briefly some of the central findings in the recent literature on the social determinants of health. If we look at cross-national studies, we see that a country's prosperity is related to its health, as measured, for example, by life expectancy: In richer countries, people tend to live longer. But the relationship between per capita gross domestic product (GDPpc) and life expectancy levels off at around $8,000 to $10,000; beyond this threshold, further economic advance buys virtually no further gains in life expectancy. This leveling effect is most apparent among the advanced industrial economies. Nevertheless, even within this relationship, there are telling variations. Though Cuba and Iraq are equally poor (each has a GDPpc of about $3,100), life expectancy in Cuba exceeds that in Iraq by 17.2 years. The poor state of Kerala in India, which invested heavily in education, especially female literacy, has health outcomes far superior to the rest of India and more comparable to those in much wealthier countries. The difference between the GDPpc for Costa Rica and the United States is enormous (about $21,000), yet Costa Rica's life expectancy exceeds that of the United States (76.6 to 76.4).

Taken together, these observations show that the health of nations depends, in part, on factors other than wealth. Culture, social organization, and government policies also help determine population health. Variations in these factors—not fixed laws of economic development—may explain many of the differences in health outcomes among nations.

One especially important factor in explaining the health of a society is the distribution of income: the health of a population depends not just on the size of the economic pie, but also on how the pie is shared. Differences in health outcomes among developed nations cannot be explained simply by the absolute deprivation associated with low economic development—lack of access to the basic material conditions necessary for health, such as clean water, adequate nutrition and housing, and general sanitary living conditions. The degree of relative deprivation within a society also matters.

Numerous studies support this *relative-income hypothesis*, which states, more precisely, that inequality is strongly associated with population mortality and life expectancy across nations (Wilkinson 1992, 1994, 1996). Rich countries vary in life expectancy, and that variation dovetails with income distribution. In particular, wealthier countries with more equal income distributions, such as Sweden and Japan, have higher life expectancies than the United States, despite having lower per capita GDP. Likewise, countries with low GDPpc but remarkably high life expectancy, such as Costa Rica, tend to have a more equitable distribution of income.

We find a similar pattern when we compare states within the United States. If we control for differences in state wealth, income inequality accounts for about 25% of the between-state variation in age-adjusted mortality rates (Kennedy, Kawachi, and Prothow-Stith 1996; Kawachi et al. 1997). Furthermore, a recent study across U.S. metropolitan areas found that areas with high income inequality had an excess of death compared to areas with low inequality—a very large excess, equivalent in magnitude to all deaths due to heart disease (Lynch et at. 1998). Longitudinal studies, which look at a single place over time and examine widening income differentials, support similar conclusions.

At the individual level we also find that inequality is important. Numerous studies have documented what has come to be known as the socioeconomic gradient: At each step along the economic ladder, we see improved health outcomes over the rung below (even in societies with universal health insurance). Differences in health outcomes are not confined to the extremes of rich and poor, but are observed across all levels of socioeconomic status.

The slope of the socioeconomic gradient varies substantially across societies. Some societies show a relatively shallow gradient in mortality rates: Being better off confers a health advantage, but not so large an advantage as elsewhere. Others, with comparable or even higher levels of economic development, show much steeper gradients. The slope of the gradient appears to be fixed by the level of income inequality in a society. The more unequal a society is in economic terms, the more unequal it is in health terms. Moreover, middle income groups in a country with high income inequality typically do worse in terms of health than comparable or even poorer groups in a society with less income inequality. We find the same pattern within the United States when we examine state and metropolitan area variations in inequality and health outcomes (Kennedy et at. 1998; Lynch et al. 1998).

Earlier, I cautioned that correlations between inequality and health do not necessarily imply causation. Still, there are enough plausible and identifiable pathways through which social inequalities appear to produce health inequalities to make a reasonable case for causation. In the United States the states with the most unequal income distributions invest less in public education, have larger uninsured populations, and spend less on social safety nets (Kaplan et al. 1996; Kawachi and Kennedy 1997). Studies of educational spending and educational outcomes are especially striking. Controlling for median income, income inequality explains about 40% of the variation between states in the percentage of children in the fourth grade who are below the basic reading level. Similarly strong associations are seen for high school drop-out rates. It is evident from these data that educational opportunities for children in high income inequality states are quite different from those in states with more egalitarian distributions. These effects on education have an immediate impact on health, increasing the likelihood of premature death during childhood and adolescence (as evidenced by the much higher death rates for infants and children in the high inequality states). Later in life these effects appear in the socioeconomic gradient in health.

When we compare countries, we also find that differential investment in human capital—in particular, education—is a strong predictor of health. Indeed, one of the strongest predictors of life expectancy among developing countries is adult literacy, particularly the disparity between male and female adult literacy, which explains much of the variation in health achievement among these countries after accounting for GDPpc. For example, among the 125 developing countries with GDPpcs of less than $10,000, the difference between male and female literacy accounts for 40% of the variation in life expectancy (after factoring out the effect of GDPpc). In the United States differences among the states in women's status—measured in terms of economic autonomy and political participation—are strongly correlated with higher female mortality rates.

These societal mechanisms—for example, income inequality leading to educational inequality leading to health inequality—are tightly linked to the political processes that influence government policy. For example, income inequality appears to affect health by undermining civil society. Income inequality erodes social cohesion, as measured by higher levels of social mistrust and reduced participation in civic organizations. Lack of social cohesion leads to lower participation in political activity (such as voting, serving in local government, volunteering for political campaigns). And lower participation, in turn, undermines the responsiveness of government institutions in addressing the needs of the worst off. States with the highest income inequality, and thus lowest levels of social capital and political participation, are less likely to invest in human capital and provide far less generous social safety nets (Kawachi and Kennedy 1999).

Rawls's principles of justice thus turn out to regulate the key social determinants of health. One principle assures equal basic liberties, and specifically provides for guaranteeing *effective* rights of political participation. The fair equality opportunity principle assures access to high quality public education, early childhood interventions (including day care) aimed at eliminating class or race disadvantages, and universal coverage for appropriate healthcare. Rawls's "Difference Principle" permits inequalities in income only if the inequalities work (e.g., through incentives) to make those who are worst off as well off as possible. This principle is not a simple "trickle down" principle that tolerates any inequality so long as there is some benefit that flows down the socioeconomic ladder; it requires a maximal flow downward. It would therefore flatten socioeconomic inequalities in a robust way, assuring far more than a "decent minimum" (Cohen 1989). In addition, the assurances of the value of political participation and fair equality of opportunity would further constrain allowable income inequalities.

The conjecture is that a society complying with these principles of justice would probably flatten the socioeconomic gradient even more than we see in the most egalitarian welfare states of northern Europe. The implication is that we should view health inequalities that derive from social determinants as unjust unless the determinants are distributed in conformity with these robust principles. Because of the detailed attention Rawls's theory pays to the interaction of these terms of fair cooperation, it provides us—through the findings of social science—with an account of the just distribution of health.

The inequalities in the social determinants that are still permitted by this theory may produce a socioeconomic gradient, albeit a much flatter one than we see today. Should we view these residual health inequalities as unjust and demand further redistribution of the social determinants?

I believe the theory I have described does not give a clear answer. If the Rawlsian theory insists that protecting opportunity takes priority over other matters and cannot be traded for other gains (and Rawls generally adopts this view), then residual health inequalities may be unjust. If health can be traded for other goods—and all of us make such trades when we take chances with our health to pursue other goals—then the account may be more flexible (Daniels, Kennedy, and Kawachi 1999). Still, Rawls's principles give us more specific guidance in thinking about the distribution of the social determinants than is given by the fair equality of opportunity account of just healthcare alone.

I noted earlier that there is considerable convergence between the opportunity-based view I defend and A. K. Sen's (1992) appeal to a capabilities-based account (or freedom based account) of the target of justice. The convergence is even more pronounced when Sen (1999) discusses the ways in which health in developing countries is affected by different development strategies and emphasizes the importance of education and the growth of democratic culture and institutions. Rawls's focus on the "capabilities of free and equal citizens" suggests the convergence works in both directions (Daniels 2000a). Both approaches allow us to talk informatively about justice and the distribution of health.

WHEN ARE LIMITS TO HEALTHCARE FAIR?

Justice requires that all societies meet healthcare needs fairly under reasonable resource constraints. Even a wealthy, egalitarian country with a highly efficient healthcare system will have to set limits to the healthcare it guarantees everyone (whether or not it allows supplementary tiers for those who can afford them). Poorer countries have to make even harder choices about priorities and limits. However important, healthcare is not the only important social good. All societies must decide which needs should be given priority and when resources are better spent elsewhere.

How should fair decisions about such limits be made? Under what conditions should we view such decisions as a legitimate exercise of moral authority?

Answering these questions would be much simpler if people could agree on principles of distributive justice that would determine how to set fair limits to healthcare. If societies agreed on such principles, people could simply check social decisions and practices against the principles to see if they conformed with them. Where decisions, practices, and institutions fail to conform, they would be unjust and people should then change them. Disagreements about the fairness of actual distributions would then be either disagreements about the interpretation of the principles or about the facts of the situation. Many societies have well-established and reliable, if imperfect, legal procedures for resolving such disputes about facts and interpretations.

Unfortunately, there is no consensus on such distributive principles for healthcare. Reasonable people, who have diverse moral and religious views about many matters, disagree morally about what constitutes a fair allocation of resources to meet competing healthcare needs—even when they agree on other aspects of the justice of healthcare systems, such as the importance of universal access to whatever services are provided. We should expect, and respect, such diversity in views about rationing healthcare. Nevertheless, we must arrive at acceptable social policies despite our disagreements. This moral controversy raises a distinctive problem of legitimacy: Under what conditions should we accept as legitimate the moral authority of those making rationing decisions?

I shall develop the following argument:

1. We have no consensus on principled solutions to a family of morally controversial rationing problems, and general principles of justice for health and healthcare fail to give specific guidance about how to solve them (Daniels 1993);
2. In the absence of such a consensus, we should rely on a fair process for arriving at solutions to these problem and for establishing the legitimacy of rationing decisions (Rawls 1971); and
3. A fair process that addresses issues of legitimacy will have to meet several constraints that I shall refer to as "accountability for reasonableness" (Daniels and Sabin 1998a); these constraints tie the process to deliberative democratic procedures (Daniels and Sabin 1997, n.d.). This issue of legitimacy and fair process arises in both public and mixed public-private healthcare systems and it must be addressed in countries at all levels of development.

To support the first step of the argument, consider a problem that has been labeled the "priorities problem" (Daniels 1993; Kamm 1993): How much priority should we give to treating the sickest or most disabled patients? To start with, imagine two extreme positions. The Maximin position ("maximize the minimum") says that we should give complete priority to treating the worst off patients. One might think that Maximin is implied by the fair equality of opportunity account (though I believe my account is only committed to giving *some* priority to the worst off, placing it in a broad family of views that leave the degree of priority unspecified). The Maximize position says that we should give priority to whatever treatment produces the greatest net health benefit (or greatest net health benefit per dollar spent) regardless of which patients we treat.

Suppose comparable resources could be invested in Technologies A or B, but the resources are "lumpy" (we cannot introduce some A and some B), and we can only afford one of A or B in our healthcare budget. The Maximin position would settle the matter by determining whether patients treated by A are worse off before treatment than patients treated by B. If so, we introduce A; if patients treated by B are worse off, we introduce B. If the two sets of patients are equally badly off, we can break the tie by considering to whom we can provide the most benefit. The Maximize position chooses between A and B solely by reference to which produces greatest net benefit.

In practice, most people are likely to reject both extreme positions (Nord 1995, 1999). If the benefits A and B produce are nearly equal, but patients needing A start off much worse than patients needing B, most people seem to believe we should introduce A. They prefer to provide A even if they know we could produce somewhat more net health benefit by introducing B. But if the net benefit produced by A is very small, or if B produces significantly more net benefit, then most people will overcome their concern to give priority to the worst off and will prefer to introduce B to A. Some people who would give priority to patients needing A temper their preference if those patients end up faring much better than patients needing B. Disagreement persists: A definite but very small, minority are inclined to be maximizers and a definite but very small minority are inclined to be maximiners. Most people fall in between, and they vary considerably in how much benefit they are willing to sacrifice in order to give priority to worse off patients.

Two other types of rationing problems also suggest we are not straight maximizers or maximiners, though we lack principled characterizations of acceptable middle-course solutions (Daniels 1993). The Fair Chances/Best Outcomes problem asks, "Should we give all who might benefit some chance at a resource, or should we give the resource to those who get the best outcome?" The Aggregation problem asks, "When do lesser benefits to many outweigh greater benefits to a few?"

Two strategies have been pursued to address these kinds of rationing problems, one philosophical, one empirical. The philosophical approach, brilliantly exemplified by Kamm's work (1993), examines subtly varied hypothetical cases, seeking to reveal agreement on a complex set of underlying principles that can account for the judgments the philosophical inquirer makes about these cases.[6] This strategy may well help us arrive at middle-level principles for addressing these rationing problems, and it should be pursued by others. Nevertheless, given the subtlety of the method and the likelihood that some disagreements about cases will reflect broader moral disagreements about other matters, I do not believe this method will produce consensus on such principles in the foreseeable future. The insights from this approach are important inputs into a fair, deliberative process of decision making, but they are not a substitute for such a fair process.

The empirical approach has been ingeniously developed by the economist Erik Nord (1999), who also explores hypothetical cases by asking groups of people "person-tradeoff" questions. These questions are a variation on a standard economic approach seeking "indifference" points or curves reflecting when an individual finds two benefits or outcomes equivalent. For example, if we can invest only in treatments A and B, and A is used for people more seriously ill than B, we might ask how many treatments with B someone would trade for some number of treatments with A. Nord hopes this approach can uncover the structure of moral concerns in a population of people. A key risk of the method is that it disguises moral disagreement by talking about a "range" of responses. For this, and other reasons I discuss elsewhere (Daniels 1998c, 2000b), the results of Nord's work can help inform fair, deliberative decision processes but cannot substitute for them.

If we have persistent disagreements about principles for resolving rationing problems, then we must retreat to a process all can agree is a fair way to resolve disputes. The retreat to procedural justice as a way of determining what is fair when we lack prior agreement on principles is a central feature of Rawls's account (thus "justice as [procedural] fairness"). Rather than argue for this familiar approach (the second step of my argument above), I shall move directly to characterizing the features of such a fair process.

We would take a giant step toward solving the problems of legitimacy and fairness that face public agencies and private health plans making limiting decisions if the following four conditions were satisfied (Daniels and Sabin 1997).[7]

Publicity Condition: Decisions regarding coverage for new technologies (and other limit-setting decisions) and their rationales must be publicly accessible.

Relevance Condition: The rationales for coverage decisions should aim to provide a *reasonable* construal of how the organization (or society) should provide "value for money" in meeting the varied health needs of a defined population under reasonable resource constraints. Specifically, a construal will be "reasonable" if it appeals to reasons and principles that are accepted as relevant by people who are disposed to finding terms of cooperation that are mutually justifiable.

Appeals Condition: There is a mechanism for challenge and dispute resolution regarding limit-setting decisions, including the opportunity for revising decisions in light of further evidence or arguments.

Enforcement Condition: There is either voluntary or public regulation of the process to ensure that conditions 1–3 are met.

The guiding idea behind the four conditions is to convert private health plan or public agency decisions into part of a larger public deliberation about how to use limited resources to protect fairly the health of a population with varied needs. The broader public deliberation envisioned here is not necessarily an organized democratic procedure, though it could include the deliberation underlying public regulation of the healthcare system. Rather, it may take place in various forms in an array of institutions, spilling over into legislative politics only under some circumstances. Meeting these conditions also serves an educative function. The public is made familiar with the need for limits and appropriate ways to reason about them.

The first condition requires that rationales for decisions be publicly accessible to all affected by them. One American health plan, for example, decided to cover growth hormone treatment, but only for children who are growth hormone deficient or who have Turner's syndrome. It deliberated carefully and clearly about the reasons for its decision. These included the lack of evidence of efficacy or good risk/benefit ratios for other groups of patients, and a commitment to restrict coverage to the treatment of disease and disability (as opposed to enhancements), It did not, however, state these reasons in its medical director's letter to clinicians or in support materials used in "shared decision making" with patients and families about the procedure. It's (sic) reasons were defensible ones aimed at a public good all can understand and see as relevant, the provision of effective and safe treatment to a defined population under resource constraints. The restriction to treatment rather than enhancement requires a moral argument, however, and remains a point about which reasonable people can disagree, as we saw earlier.

One important effect of making public the reasons for coverage decisions is that, over time, the pattern of such decisions will resemble a type of "case law." A body of case law establishes the presumption that if some individuals have been treated one way because they fall under a reasonable interpretation of the relevant principles, then similar individuals should be treated the same way in subsequent cases. In effect, the institution generating the case law is saying, "We deliberate carefully about hard cases and have good reasons for doing what we have done, and we continue to stand by our reasons in our commitment to act consistently with past practices." To rebut this presumption requires showing either that the new case differs in relevant and important ways from the earlier one, justifying different treatment, or that there are good grounds for rejecting the reasons or principles embodied in the earlier case. Case law does not imply past infallibility, but it does imply giving careful consideration to why earlier decision makers made the choices they did. It involves a form of institutional reflective equilibrium, a commitment to both transparency and coherence in the giving of reasons.

The benefits of publicity in the form of case law are both internal and external to the decision-making institution. The quality of decision making improves if reasons must be articulated. Fairness improves over time, both formally, since like cases are treated similarly, and substantively, since there is systematic evaluation of reasons. To the extent that we are then better able to discover flaws in our moral reasoning, we are more likely to arrive at fair decisions. Over time, people will understand better the moral commitments of the institutions making these decisions.

The Relevance Condition imposes two important constraints on the rationales that are made publicly accessible. Specifically, the rationales for coverage decisions should aim to provide (a) a *reasonable* construal of (b) how the organization (or society) should provide "value for money" in meeting the varied health needs of a defined population under reasonable resource limits. Both constraints need explanation.

We may think of the goal of meeting the varied needs of the population of patients under reasonable resource constraints as a characterization of the *common or public good* pursued by all engaged in the enterprise of delivering and receiving this care. Reasoning about that goal must also meet certain conditions. Specifically, a construal of the goal will be "reasonable" only if it appeals to reasons (evidence, values, and principles) that are accepted as relevant by "fair-minded" people. By "fair-minded" I mean people who seek mutually justifiable terms of cooperation. The notion is not mysterious, since we encounter it all the time in sports. Fair-minded people are those who want to play by agreed-upon rules in a sport and prefer rules that are designed to bring out the best in that game. Here we are concerned with the game of delivering healthcare that meets population needs in a fair way.

Recall the restriction on the use of growth hormone treatment to those with growth hormone deficiency. As I noted earlier, some object that a theory that emphasizes protecting equal opportunity, as mine does, should also use medical interventions to eliminate extreme but normal shortness if it is disadvantaging. Still, proponents on both sides of this dispute can recognize that reasonable people might disagree about the specific requirements of a principle protecting opportunity. Both sides of the dispute about the scope of the goals of medicine nevertheless must recognize the relevance and appropriateness of the kind of reason offered by the other, even if they disagree with the interpretation of the principle or the applications to which it is put.

Consider further the implications of the Relevance Condition. "Including this treatment befits me (and other patients like me)," just like "excluding this treatment disadvantages me (or other patients like me)," is not the kind of reason that meets the constraints on reasons. Because comparative coverage decisions always advantage some and disadvantage others, mere advantage or disadvantage is not a relevant reason in debates about coverage. If, however, a coverage decision disadvantages me compared to other patients similar to me in all relevant ways, then this is reason based on disadvantage that all must think is relevant. Also, if a coverage decision disadvantages someone (and others like him or her) more than anyone need be disadvantaged under alternatives available, then this too is a reason that all must consider relevant.

How should we view the claim that a treatment "costs too much"? First, suppose this is a claim about relative cost-effectiveness or worthiness. People who share in the goal of meeting the varied medical needs of a population covered by limited resources would consider relevant the claim that a particular technology falls below some defensible threshold of cost-effectiveness or relative cost-worthiness. Suppose, however, the claim that something "costs too much" refers to its effects on profits or competitiveness. Supporting this claim often requires providing information that private health plans will not reveal (for good business reasons), often turns on economic and strategic judgments requiring special experience and training, and ultimately depends on a much more fundamental claim about the design of the system, namely, that a system involving competition in this sort of market will produce efficiencies that work to the advantage of all who have medical needs. My point is not that these reasons fail to meet the Relevance Condition, but that providing support for them requires information that is often not available, that is hard to understand when it is available, and that ultimately depends on fundamental moral and political judgments about the feasibility of quite different alternative systems for delivering healthcare. Nevertheless, if for-profit health plans are to comply with the Relevance Condition, they must either be willing to provide information they would ordinarily not make public, or make their decisions on the basis of reasons that they can defend to other relevant stakeholders.

The constraints here imposed on reasons have a bearing on a philosophical debate about the legitimacy of democratic procedures. An aggregative or proceduralist conception of democratic voting sees it as a way of aggregating preferences. Where, however, we are concerned with fundamental differences in values, not mere preferences, an aggregative view seems inadequate. It seems insensitive to how we ideally would like to resolve moral disputes, namely through argument and deliberation. An alternative "deliberative" view imposes constraints on the kinds of reasons that can play a role in de-liberation. Not just any preferences will do. Reasons must reflect the fact that all parties to a decision are viewed as seeking terms of fair cooperation that they accept as reasonable. Even if we have to rely on a majority vote to set-tle a disagreement where there are serious moral issues involved, if the rea-sons are constrained to those all must view as relevant, then the minority can at least assure itself that the preference of the majority rests on the kind of rea-son that even the minority must acknowledge appropriately plays a role in de-liberation. The majority does not exercise brute power of preference but is in-stead constrained by having to seek reasons for its view that are justifiable to all who seek mutually justifiable terms of cooperation.

The Appeals and Enforcement Conditions involve mechanisms that go be-yond the publicity requirements of the first two conditions. When patients or clinicians use these procedures to challenge a decision, and the results of the challenge lead effectively to reconsideration of the decision on its merits, the decision-making process is made iterative in a way that broadens the input of information and argument. Parties that were excluded from the decision-making process, and whose views may not have been clearly heard or under-stood, find a voice, even if after the original fact. The dispute resolution mechanisms do not empower enrollees or clinicians to play a direct, partici-patory role in the actual decision-making bodies, but that does not happen in many public democratic processes either. Still, it does empower them to play a more effective role in the larger social deliberation about the issues, includ-ing in those public institutions that can play a role in regulating private health plans or otherwise constraining their acts. The mechanisms we describe thus play a role in assuring broader accountability of private organizations to those who are affected by limit-setting decisions. The arrangements required by the four conditions provide connective tissue to, not a replacement for, broader democratic processes that ultimately have authority and responsibility for guaranteeing the fairness of limit setting decisions.

Together these conditions hold institutions—public or private—and deci-sion makers in them "accountable for the reasonableness" of the limits they set. All must engage in a process of establishing their credentials for fair deci-sion making about such fundamental matters every time they make such a de-cision. Whether in public or mixed systems, establishing the accountability of decision makers to those affected by their decisions is the only way to show, over time, that arguably fair decisions are being made and that those making them have established a procedure we should view as legitimate. This is not to say that public participation is an essential ingredient of the process in either public or mixed systems, but the accountability to the public in both cases is necessary to facilitate broader democratic processes that regulate the system.

In many public systems the reasoning that lies behind decisions that affect the length of queues—a rationing device—are inscrutable to the public. They are made in a "black box" of budgetary decisions. Queues may then be adjusted if the public complains too much—there is this kind of accountability to the squeaky wheel. But there is in general too little accountability of the sort demanded by the four conditions I describe (Ham and Packard 1998; Coulter and Ham 2000). Only through such accountability and the way in which it facilitates or enables a broader social deliberation will there be a wider perception that rationing decisions are fair and are made through an exercise of legitimate authority.

One issue facing this "process" approach to rationing seem to be more problematic in public systems than it does in mixed ones. In a mixed system two different insurers or health plans might arrive at different judgments about what limits to set. I have suggested both might be "right" if their decisions are the results of fair procedures (Daniels and Sabin 1998b). The anomaly is that some patients will then have access to services that others will not have, and this might seem to violate a formal constraint on fairness, that society treat like cases similarly. In a mixed system we might see this variation as a price we pay for whatever virtues (if any) the mixed system brings (the variation might ultimately lead us to better decisions over time). In a public system, however, such variation, e.g., between districts, might seem more objectionable if all are governed by the same public legislation and funding. Still, despite such anomalies, fair process may be the best we can do wherever we have no prior consensus on fair outcomes.

CONCLUDING REMARKS

A comprehensive approach to justice, health and healthcare must address all three questions I have discussed. My extension of Rawls's theory of justice to health and healthcare provides a way to link answers to the first and second questions. There are three ways in which Rawls's theory also provides support for my approach to the third question. First, I propose that we use a fair process to arrive at what is fair in rationing, since we lack prior consensus on the relevant distributive principles. This retreat to procedural justice is at the heart of Rawls's own invocation of his version of a social contract. Second, Rawls places great emphasis on the importance of publicity as a constraint on theories of justice. Principles of justice and the grounds for them must be publicly acknowledged. This constraint is central to the conditions that establish accountability for reasonableness. Finally, Rawls develops the view that "public reason" must constrain the content of public deliberations and decisions about fundamental matters of justice, avoiding special considerations that might be elements of the comprehensive moral views that people hold (Rawls 1993). Accountability for reasonableness pushes decision makers toward finding reasons all can agree are relevant to the goals of cooperative health delivery schemes. In this way accountability for reasonableness promotes the democratic deliberation that Rawls also advocates.

In pointing out these connections, I am not suggesting that this is the only approach to developing a theory of justice that applies to all aspects of health and healthcare. Indeed, I have pointed to other theories that converge in practice and to some extent in theory with the approach adopted here. I am proposing that concerns about justice and fairness in health policy should look to political philosophy for guidance and that some specific guidance is forthcoming. At the very same time, seeing how we have to modify and refine work in political philosophy if it is to apply to real issues in the world suggests that we should abandon the unidirectional implications of the term "applied ethics" or "applied political philosophy" (Daniels 1996b).

NOTES

1. Disease and disability, both physical and mental, are construed as adverse departures from or impairments of species-typical normal functional organization, or "normal functioning" for short. The line between disease and disability and normal functioning is drawn in the relatively objective and nonevaluative context provided by the biomedical sciences, broadly construed (though glaring misclassifications have also occurred). I ignore the considerable controversy in the philosophy of biology about how to analyze the concept of function (Daniels 1985).

2. Daniels (1996a) discusses the relationship between the equal opportunity account and the rationale for "reasonable accommodation" required of employers under the Americans with Disabilities Act; see also Brock (1995). Brock (1998) discusses the implication of disabilities for cost-effectiveness analysis; see also Buchanan et al. (2000), ch. 7.

3. Economists view an arrangement as efficient or pareto optimal if no one can be made better off without making someone else worse off. If some people trade their access to healthcare through socially provided insurance for other goods, they are not in a pareto optimal situation.

4. The age rationing implied by this account is different in rationale from that advocated by Callahan (1987), who thinks the old have a duty to step aside in favor of the young; it is also different from those who argue for a version of the "fair innings"

view, which gives priority to the young on the grounds that the old have already had their opportunity to acquire years (see for example, Brock 1989; Williams 1997); it is also different in rationale from Kamm (1993), who argues that the young would be worse off than the old and in that sense "need" years more than the old, The considerable disagreement about what justice permits, even among those who accept some forms of age rationing, argues for the importance of the type of fair process described later in this paper.

5. See Daniels (2000a); also Rawls (1993). The convergence is clearer still when Sen (1999) addresses the ways in which we should focus on our capabilities as citizens—see Anderson (1999).

6. Kamm insists on exploring hypothetical cases or thought experiments rather than real ones, attempting to isolate more clearly in these cases the relevant features that motivate our judgments. She believes that her method will uncover an "internal program" or underlying moral structure to our beliefs. Crucial to this approach is the claim that people will agree on a central range of cases, that is that others will have the same responses Kamm does to them. For doubts about the method, see Daniels (1998b).

7. The conditions described were developed independently but fit reasonably well with the framework of principles for democratic deliberation developed by Gutmann and Thompson (1996). For some reservations about their approach, see Daniels (1999).

ACKNOWLEDGMENTS

This article appears by agreement with and courtesy of Oxford University Press (New York, New York), and appears in *Medicine and Social Justice*, edited by Rosamond Rhodes, Margaret Pabst Battin, and Anita Silvers in 2002. Bruce Kennedy and Ichiro Kawachi collaborated with me to write the material on which I draw for the section, "Which health inequalities are unjust?" James Sabin collaborated on the research and writing on which I draw for the section, "When are limits to healthcare fair?" Research for this paper was supported by a Robert Wood Johnson Investigator Award and Tufts Sabbatical Leave. I have benefited from discussions with Richard Arneson, Allen Buchanan, Dan Brock, G. A. Cohen, Joshua Cohen, John Rawls, and Dan Wikler about the relationship between my approach and that of other recent work on egalitarianism.

REFERENCES

Acheson, D. et al. 1998. *Report of the independent inquiry into inequalities in health.* London: Stationary Office.

Anderson, E. 1999. What is the point of equality? *Ethics* 109:287–337.

Arneson, R. J. 1988. Equality and equal opportunity for welfare. *Philosophical Studies* 54:79–95.

Black, D., J. N. Morris, C. Smith, P. Townsend, and M. Whitehead. 1988. *Inequalities in health: The Black Report; The health divide.* London: Penguin Group.

Brock, D. 1989. Justice, healthcare, and the elderly. *Philosophy & Public Affairs* 18(3):297–312.

———. 1995. Justice and the ADA: Does prioritizing and rationing healthcare discriminate against the disabled? *Social Philosophy and Policy* 12:159–184.

———. 1998. Ethical issues in the development of summary measures of health status. In *Summarizing population health: Directions for the development and application of population metrics,* Institute of Medicine, Washington: National Academy Press.

Buchanan, A., D. Brock, N. Daniels, and D. Wikler. 2000. *From chance to choice: Genetics and justice.* New York: Cambridge University Press.

Callahan, D. 1987. *Setting limits: Medical goals in an aging society.* New York: Simon & Schuster.

Cohen, G. A. 1989. On the currency of egalitarian justice. *Ethics* 99:906–944.

Cohen, J. 1989. Democratic equality. *Ethics* 99:727–751.

Coulter, A., and C. Ham. 2000. *The global challenge of healthcare rationing.* Buckingham: Open University Press.

Daniels, N. 1981. Health-care needs and distributive justice. *Philosophy and Public Affairs* 10: 146–179.

———. 1985. *Just healthcare.* New York: Cambridge University Press.

———. 1988. *Am I my parents' keeper? An essay on justice between the old and the young.* New York: Oxford University Press.

———. 1990. Equality of what: Welfare, resources, or capabilities? *Philosophy and Phenomenological Research* 50(Supplement):273–296.

———. 1993. Rationing Fairly: Programmatic considerations. *Bioethics* 7(2/3):224–233. Reprinted in Daniels 1996b, 317–326.

———. 1995. *Seeking fair treatment. From the AIDS epidemic to national healthcare reform.* New York: Oxford University Press.

———. 1996a. Mental disabilities, equal opportunity, and the ADA. In *Mental disorder, work disability, and the law,* ed. R. J. Bonnie and J. Monahan, 282–297. Chicago: University of Chicago Press.

———. 1996b. *Justice and justification: Reflective equilibrium in theory and practice.* New York: Cambridge University Press.

———. 1998a. Rationing medical care: A philosopher's perspective on outcomes and process. *Economics and Philosophy* 14:27–50.

———. 1998b. Kamm's moral methods. *Philosophy and Phenomenological Research* 58(4):947–954.

———. 1998c. Distributive justice and the use of summary measures of population health status. In *Summarizing population health: Directions for the development and application of population metrics,* Institute of Medicine, 58– 71. Washington: National Academy Press.

———. 1999. Enabling democratic deliberation: How managed care organizations ought to make decisions about coverage for new technologies. In *Deliberative politics. Essays on democracy and disagreement,* ed. S. Macedo, 198–210. New York: Oxford University Press.

24 *Daniels*

——. 2000a. Democratic equality: Rawls's complex egalitarianism. In *Companion to Rawls*, ed. S. Freeman. Oxford: Blackwells, forthcoming.

——. 2000b. Legitimacy, fair process, and limits to healthcare. World Health Organization Project on Fairness and Goodness, forthcoming.

Daniels, N., B. Kennedy, and I. Kawachi. 1999. Why justice is good for our health: Social determinants of health inequalities. *Daedalus* 128(4):215–251.

Daniels, N., B. Kennedy, I. Kawachi, and A. Sen. 2000. *Is inequality bad for our health?* Boston: Beacon Press.

Daniels, N., D. Light, and R. Caplan. 1996. *Benchmarks of fairness for healthcare reform.* New York: Oxford University Press.

Daniels, N., and J. E. Sabin. 1997. Limits to healthcare: Fair procedures, democratic deliberation, and the legitimacy problem for insurers. *Philosophy and Public Affairs* 26:303–350.

——. 1998a. The ethics of accountability and the reform of managed care organizations. *Health Affairs* 17(5):50–69.

——. 1998b. Last-chance therapies and managed care: Pluralism, fair procedures, and legitimacy. *Hastings Center Report* 28(2):27–41.

——. 2001. *Setting limits fairly: Can we learn to share medical resources?* New York: Oxford University Press, forthcoming.

Gutmann, A., and D. Thompson. 1996. *Democracy and disagreement.* Cambridge: Harvard University Press.

Ham, C., and S. Pickard. 1998. *Tragic choices in healthcare: The story of Child B.* London: Kings Fund.

Kamm, F. M. 1993. Morality, mortality. *Vol 1: Death and whom to save from it.* Oxford: Oxford University Press.

Kaplan, G. A., E. R. Pamuk, J. W. Lynch et al. 1996. Inequality in income and mortality in the United States: Analysis of mortality and potential pathways. *British Medical Journal* 312:999–1003.

Kawachi, I., and B. P. Kennedy. 1997. Health and social cohesion: Why care about income inequality? *British Medical Journal* 314:1037–1040.

——. 1999. Income inequality and health: Pathways and mechanisms. *Health Services Research* 34:215–227.

Kawachi, I., B. P. Kennedy, and R. Wilkinson, eds. 1999. *Income inequality and health: A reader.* New York: The New Press.

Kawachi, I., B. P. Kennedy, K. Lochner, and D. Prothrow-Stith. 1997. Social capital, income inequality, and mortality. *American Journal of Public Health* 87:1491–1498.

Kennedy, B. P., I. Kawachi, R. Glass, and D. Prothrow-Stith. 1998. Income distribution, socioeconomic status, and self-rated health: A U.S. multi-level analysis. *British Medical Journal* 317:917–921.

Kennedy, B. P., I. Kawachi, and D. Prothrow-Stith. 1996. Income distribution and mortality: Test of the Robin Hood Index in the United States. *British Medical Journal* 312:1004–1008. Published erratum appears in *British Medical Journal* 312:1194.

Kennedy, B. P., I. Kawachi, D. Prothrow-Stith, and V. Gupta. 1998. Income inequality, social capital, and firearm-related violent crime. *Social Science and Medicine* 47:7–17.

Lynch, J. W., G. A. Kaplan, E. R. Pamuk et al. 1998. Income inequality and mortality in metropolitan areas of the United States. *American Journal of Public Health* 88:1074–1080.

Marmot, M. G. 1999. Social causes of social inequalities in health. Harvard Center for Population and Development Studies, Working Paper. Series 99.01, January 1999.

Marmot, M. G., R. Fuhrer, S. L. Ettner et al. 1998. Contribution of psychosocial factors to socioeconomic differences in health. *Milbank Quarterly* 76(3):403–448.

Nord, E. 1995. The person-tradeoff approach to valuing healthcare programs. *Medical Decision Making* 15:201–208.

———. 1999. *Cost-value analysis in healthcare: Making sense out of QALYS*. Cambridge: Cambridge University Press.

Rawls, J. 1971. *A theory of justice*. Cambridge: Harvard University Press.

———. 1993. *Political liberalism*. New York: Columbia University Press.

Sabin, J., and N. Daniels. 1994. Determining 'medical necessity' in mental health practice: A study of clinical reasoning and a proposal for insurance policy. *Hasting Center Reports* 24(6):5–13.

Scanlon, T. M. 1975. Preference and urgency. *Journal of Philosophy* 77 (19):655–669.

Sen, A. K. 1980. Equality of what? In *Tanner Lectures on human values*, vol 1, ed. S. McMurrin. Cambridge: Cambridge University Press.

———. 1992. Inequality reexamined. Cambridge: Harvard University Press.

———. 1999. *Development as freedom*. New York: Alfred A. Knopf.

Wilkinson, R. G. 1992. Income distribution and life expectancy. *British Medical Journal* 304:165–168.

———. 1994. The epidemiological transition: From material scarcity to social disadvantage? *Daedalus* 123:61–77.

———. 1996. *Unhealthy societies: The afflictions of inequality*. London: Routledge.

Williams, A. 1997. Intergenerational equity: An exploration of the 'fair innings' argument. *Health Economics* 6:117–132.

2

An Unequal Epidemic in an Unequal World

Kevin M. De Cock and Robert S. Janssen

In July 2002, approximately 15,000 clinicians, researchers, and other interested persons gathered once again, this time at the XIV International AIDS Conference in Barcelona, to discuss what is arguably the worst plague the world has ever known. These international conferences and their venues are milestones in the history of this tragic epidemic. In 1985, Atlanta hosted the first meeting; in 1996, the Vancouver meeting introduced combination therapy and viral load testing to the world; and in 2000, Durban drew international attention to Africa's plight. Barcelona offered further opportunity for dialogue, reflection on epidemiology and response, and strengthening global resolve.

The United States is the most heavily affected country in the industrialized world with almost 1 million persons living with HIV (human immunodeficiency virus).[1] Important successes have included the prevention of HIV/AIDS (acquired immunodeficiency syndrome) transmitted through blood and blood products; progress toward elimination of pediatric HIV disease as a result of prevention of mother-to-child transmission of HIV; and reductions in AIDS incidence and deaths since 1996 through use of highly active antiretroviral therapy (HAART); however, the trend in incidence and death has now stabilized.[2]

Despite some advances, HIV incidence in the United States has not declined significantly over the past decade, with approximately 40000 new infections occurring annually.[1] Unfortunately, HIV infection continues to affect disproportionately communities of color, especially African Americans.[1,2] Moreover, with unchanged incidence and longer survival, a slow increase has occurred in the total number of persons living with HIV. Because HAART has delayed the development of AIDS, back calculation, a technique used to

27

model HIV incidence from AIDS case surveillance data,[3] is no longer possible. Of note, in part because of the successes of HAART, there has been a recent resurgence of unsafe behavior among men who have sex with men (MSM), resulting in well-characterized outbreaks of sexually transmitted infections such as syphilis, and, perhaps, increased HIV transmission.[4,5]

Three public health priorities for the United States are: (1) to refashion the national HIV/AIDS surveillance system to focus on HIV[6] and obtain insight into HIV incidence; (2) to reinvigorate prevention efforts nationally; and (3) to promote prevention specifically among HIV-infected persons to prevent onward transmission.[7] Among MSM and other populations with high rates of HIV/AIDS, emphasis must be placed on voluntary counseling and testing, medical evaluation and care, prevention services for HIV-infected individuals, and adoption of the philosophy of personal responsibility not to transmit HIV.

The joint United Nations Programme on HIV/AIDS (UNAIDS) estimated that in late 2001 approximately 40 million persons worldwide were living with HIV/AIDS, that 5 million new HIV infections occurred in that year, and that 3 million HIV-infected persons died.[8] In Central and South America, MSM and injecting drug users account for the majority of infected persons in most countries.[8] In western Europe,[9] HIV/AIDS has become endemic, despite major differences between different countries. In some European countries heterosexual transmission now accounts for the majority of new HIV infections,[9] although a substantial proportion of newly reported infections are imported, especially from Africa.[9]

The most unpredictable epidemiological situations are in eastern Europe and Asia. Extensive HIV testing has been conducted in eastern Europe, but there have been few systematic prevalence studies.[9] The majority of HIV infections are (sic) associated with injecting drug use and occur in men; the male to female ratio of reported infections is more than 3 to 1.[9] The number of new infections in the last few years has increased steeply in Ukraine, the Russian Federation, Latvia, and Estonia, but spread is now occurring throughout most of the region.[9] Eastern Europe needs better surveillance data, interventions to reduce drug use and needle and syringe sharing, and prevention of secondary sexual spread of HIV.

Transmission of HIV in Asia remains largely restricted to injection drug users and commercial sex workers and their clients, with secondary sexual transmission from these core groups to their steady partners.[8] Generalized heterosexual spread as seen in Africa has not occurred, and vigorous efforts in Thailand to achieve universal condom use in commercial sex settings had rapid impact on decreasing HIV transmission.[10] Although the situation in the 2 most populous countries, India and China, is unclear, the prevalence of HIV infection among pregnant women, still the most useful sentinel population, has remained well below 5% in most of the region.[11] India is estimated to have 4 million HIV-infected persons.[11] China's epidemic is predominantly associated with injection drug use, and HIV prevalence levels of 70% or more have been reported among drug injectors in some areas.[11] Evidence of extensive HIV infection in rural Henan Province in central China has emerged and is related to unsterile practices in the commercial blood trade.[11] Focusing prevention efforts on injection drug use and commercial sex, and ensuring a safe blood transfusion infrastructure, will help prevent the greatest number of new HIV infections in Asia. What happens in this most populous continent, especially in India and China, will profoundly influence the future history of the HIV/AIDS pandemic.

In Africa, where HIV/AIDS is generalized, the epidemic is uniquely severe. Of the world burden of HIV infection, the sub-Saharan Africa region represents 77% of AIDS deaths, 70% of HIV-infected persons, and 68% of new infections.[8] The region has more than 90% of the children with HIV infection and AIDS orphans in the world.[8] Antenatal HIV prevalence is greater than 10% in more than a dozen cities in sub-Saharan Africa, and in some it exceeds 20% and even 30%.[12] In many countries the probability that an adolescent will ultimately die of AIDS is greater than 50%.[13] The impact of HIV/AIDS on all sectors of society is unlike that associated with any other disease. Extreme differences in epidemic severity are seen across the continent, with the east and southern parts most heavily affected.[12, 14]

Increased attention is now being paid to the pandemic by international political leaders, evidenced by the creation of the Global Fund to Fight AIDS, Tuberculosis and Malaria (GFATM).[15] Global health is now seen as an issue with political, economic, and security implications.[16] This increased attention and funding offer the best chance in decades to improve the health of the global poor, but formidable obstacles include the targeting of effort, adequacy of funding, technical limitations, difficulties of implementation, and the limited priority accorded to health in poor countries. Because conditions are most adverse in Africa, which lags behind the rest of the world in virtually all measures of economic and social development, Africa is the absolute test of effectiveness of interventions for HIV/AIDS and other diseases associated with poverty.

Although HIV/AIDS is the most pressing problem, there is under-recognition of the collapse of public health and clinical infrastructure in general in Africa over the past 25 years, independent of, as well as sometimes exacerbated by, HIV/AIDS. For example, chloroquine resistance has resulted in increases in malaria-related mortality in Africa during the 1990s, and resistance to sulfadoxime-pyrimethamine is also increasing.[17] Tuberculosis case rates are increasing by 10% to 15% annually in many countries largely because of HIV/AIDS.[18] Conflict has adversely affected health in numerous settings; an estimated 2.5 million excess deaths occurred in the eastern part of the Democratic Republic of the Congo over a recent 3-year period, largely from infectious diseases and malnutrition.[19] Environmental and social conditions have favored the emergence and reemergence of different infectious diseases, such as sleeping sickness in the Democratic Republic of the Congo.[20] Substantial increases in infant and under-5 mortality have occurred.[21, 22] as well as in maternal mortality, a longstanding and neglected problem.[23-25] Thus, there is evidence to suggest that a number of aspects of health status in general show decline both independent of and exacerbated by AIDS.

The Commission on Macroeconomics and Health[26] estimated that to substantially improve global health, donor funding to all low-income countries would have to increase by $27 billion by 2007, from current levels of approximately $6 billion, and by $38 billion by 2015. The call for approximately $8 billion annually for the GFATM is included in these figures. In an analysis of requirements for an expanded response to HIV/AIDS alone, Schwartlander and Colleagues[27] estimated that by 2005, $9.2 billion would be needed annually in middle- and low-income countries, with half of the resource needs represented by requirements for sub-Saharan Africa. Currently, less than $2 billion has been pledged to the GFATM.

Technical limitations concerning interventions for Africa's major health challenges also are overlooked in the enthusiasm of advocacy and fundraising. There is no uniform HIV/AIDS prevention program to roll out internationally, the efficacy of sexually transmitted disease control as an HIV prevention strategy is not entirely clear,[18] mother-to-child transmission prevention is proving more difficult programmatically than in clinical trials (Anja van't Hoog et al, unpublished data, 2002), and there is no consensus about the appropriate balance between prevention and care, or how to expand access to HAART in Africa.[28] HIV/AIDS prevention initiatives may have underemphasized the importance of HIV testing and partner notification in Africa's high prevalence, generalized epidemic.[29] As an example of limitations in successfully tackling major diseases in Africa, DOTS (directly observed therapy-short course), the tuberculosis control strategy of the World Health Organization, is failing in areas of high HIV prevalence.[30] In addition, drug resistance challenges effective antimalarial treatment, a component of the World Health Organization Roll Back Malaria program.[31] Science-based solutions to these and myriad other problems are required for the high aspirations of the GFATM to be met.

A particular challenge in Africa is to convert increased funding into better services at the local level, through what the Commission on Macroeconomics and Health referred to as "close-to-client" systems.[26] The GFATM will be judged on the degree to which enhanced prevention and clinical services affect the health of the poor. This will require linkages between industrialized and developing country governmental and other institutions and groups, and investment in rebuilding health infrastructure. In addition to enhanced preventive services, there is a need for simple, quality health care services for infectious diseases in children and adults, pregnancy and its complications, and surgical conditions, especially trauma.[32]

In conclusion, the XIV International AIDS Conference in Barcelona will be a contrast of extremes. Although the impact of AIDS is now less obvious in the industrialized world, HIV transmission continues in specific groups such as MSM, and a disproportionate burden of disease exists in underprivileged communities. The situation in the former Soviet Union epitomizes epidemic spread of HIV through injection drug use, a problem for which global control is elusive. Injection drug use and commercial sex fuel HIV transmission in Asia. Focused interventions for these focal epidemics can have great effect. The situation in Africa is different in scale and scope, with a devastating, generalized HIV/AIDS epidemic superimposed on an eroding health infrastructure burdened by other health threats. A fundamental question is to what extent public health strategies can reverse Africa's current adverse health trends without long-term economic development or an HIV vaccine. Despite the obstacles, the increased attention to and resources for global health, the moral challenge of this era, offer hope and opportunities not seen before in the history of the HIV/AIDS pandemic.

NOTES

1. Karon JM, Fleming PL, Steketee RW, De Cock KM. HIV in the United States at the turn of the century: an epidemic in transition. *Am J Public Health.* 2001;91: 1060-1068.

2. *HIV/AIDS Surveillance Report.* Atlanta, Ga: Centers for Disease Control and Prevention; 2001;13(No. 1):1-41.

3. Rosenberg PS, Biggar RJ. Trends in HIV incidence among young adults in the United States. *JAMA.* 1998;279:1894-1899.

4. Stall RD, Hays RB, Waldo CR, et al. The Gay '90s: a review of research in the 1990s on sexual behavior and HIV risk among men who have sex with men. *AIDS.* 2000;14(suppl 3):S101-S114.

5. Katz MH, Schwarcz SK, Kellogg TA, et al. Impact of highly active antiretroviral treatment on HIV seroincidence among men who have sex with men: San Francisco. *Am J Public Health.* 2002;92:388 394.

6. Centers for Disease Control and Prevention. Guidelines for human immunodeficiency virus case surveillance, including monitoring for human imunodeficiency virus infection and acquired immunodeficiency syndrome. *MM WR Morb Mortal Wkly Rep.* 1999;48(No. RR-13)1-27.

32 *De Cock and Janssen*

7. Janssen RS, Holtgrave Dr, Valdiserri RO, et al. The serostatus approach to fighting the HIV epidemic: prevention strategies for HIV-infected individuals. *Am J Public Health.* 2001;91:1019-1024.

8. UNAIDS/WHO. *AIDS Epidemic Update, December 2001.* Geneva, Switzerland: UNAIDS/WHO; 2001.

9. EuroHIV. *HIV/AIDS Surveillance in Europe.* Saint-Maurice, France: European Centre for the Epidemiological Monitoring of AIDS; 2001;65:1-61.

10. Kilmarx PH, Supawitkul S, Wankrairoj M, et al. Explosive spread and effective control of human immunodeficiency virus in northernmost Thailand: the epidemic in Chiang Rai province, 1988-1999. *AIDS.* 2000;14:2731-2740.

11. UNAIDS. Epidemiological Fact Sheets by Country. Available at: http://www.UNAIDS.org. Accessibility verified June 12, 2002.

12. *Recent HIV Seroprevalence Levels by Country: June 2001.* Washington, DC: US Bureau of The Census; 2001.

13. Zaba B. Lifetime risk of AIDS death for 15-year old boys, assuming unchanged or halved risk of becoming infected with HIV, selected countries. In: UNAIDS. *Report on the Global HIV/AIDS Epidemic, June 2000.* Geneva, Switzerland; UNAIDS/WHO; 2000:26.

14. Buve A, Carael M, Hayes RJ, et al. The multicentre study on factors determining the differential spread of HIV in four African cities: summary and conclusions. *AIDS.* 2001;15 (suppl 4):SI27-SI31.

15. The Global Fund to Fight AIDS, Tuberculosis and Malaria. Available at: http://www.globalfundatm.org. Accessibility verified June 12, 2002.

16. Central Intelligence Agency. The Global infectious Disease Threat and Its Implications for the United States. Available at: http://www.cia.gov. Accessibility verified June 12, 2002.

17. Ronn A, Msangeni HA, Mhina J, et al. High level of resistance of *Plasmodium falciparum* to sulfadoxine-pyrimethamine in children in Tanzania. *Trans R Soc Trop Med Hyg.* 1996;90:179-181.

18. Corbett EL, Steketee RW, ter Kuile F, et al. HIV/AIDS and the control of other infectious diseases in Africa. *Lancet.* 2002;359:2177-2187.

19. *Mortality in Eastern Democratic Republic of Congo: Results From Eleven Mortality Surveys.* New York, NY: International Rescue Committee; 2001.

20. Van Nieuwenhove S, Betu-Ku-Mesu VK, Diabakana PM, et al. Sleeping sickness resurgence in the DRC: the past decade. *Trop Med Int Health.* 2001;6:335-341.

21. *Kenya Demographic and Health Survey 1998.* Calverton, Md: National Council for Population and Development, Central Bureau of Statistics (Office of the Vice President and Ministry of Planning and National Development) [Kenya], and Macro International Inc; 1999.

22. McElroy PO, ter Kuile FO, Hightower AW, et al. All-cause mortality among young children in western Kenya, VI: the Asembo Bay Cohort Project. *Am J Trop Med Hyg.* 2001;64(1-2 supp])S18-S27.

23. Hill K, AbouZhar C, Wardlaw T. Estimates for maternal mortality for 1995. *Bull WHO.* 2001;79:182-193.

24. Bicego G, Boerma JT, Ronsmans C. The effect of AIDS on maternal mortality in Malawi and Zimbabwe. *AIDS*. 2002;16:1078-1081.

25. Ahmed Y, Mwaba P, Chintu C, et al. A study of maternal mortality at the University Teaching Hospital, Lusaka, Zambia: the emergence of tuberculosis as a major non-obstetric cause of maternal death. *Int J Tuberc Lung Dis*. 1999;3:675-680.

26. Commission on Macroeconomics and Health. *Macroeconornics and Health: investing in Health for Economic Development*. Geneva, Switzerland: World Health Organization; 2001.

27. Schwartlander B, Stover J, Walker N, et al. Resource needs for HIV/AIDS. *Science*. 2001;292:2434-2436.

28. Weidle PJ, Mastro TD, Grant AD, et al. HIV/AIDS treatments and HIV vaccines for Africa. *Lancet*. 2002;359:2261-2267.

29. De Cock KM, Mbori-Ngacha D, Marum E. Shadow on the continent: public health and HIV/AIDS in Africa in the 21st century. *Lancet*. 2002;360:67-72.

30. DeCock KM, Chaisson RE. Will DOTS do it? a reappraisal of tuberculosis control in countries with high rates of HIV infection. *lnt J Tuberc Lung Dis*. 1999;3:457-465.

31. White NJ, Nosten F, Looareesuwan S, et al. Averting a malaria disaster. *Lancet*. 1999;353:1965-1967.

32. World Bank. *World Development Report 1993: Investing in Health*. Oxford, England: Oxford University Press; 1993.

3

The Importance of Race and Ethnic Background in Biomedical Research and Clinical Practice

Esteban González Burchard, Elad Ziv, Natasha Coyle,
Scarlett Lin Gomez, Hua Tang, Andrew J. Karter,
Joanna L. Mountain, Eliseo J. Pérez-Stable,
Dean Sheppard, and Neil Risch

A debate has recently arisen over the use of racial classification in medicine and biomedical research. In particular, with the completion of a rough draft of the human genome, some have suggested that racial classification may not be useful for biomedical studies, since it reflects "a fairly small number of genes that describe appearance"[1] and "there is no basis in the genetic code for race."[2] In part on the basis of these conclusions, some have argued for the exclusion of racial and ethnic classification from biomedical research.[3] In the United States, race and ethnic background have been used as cause for discrimination, prejudice, marginalization, and even subjugation. Excessive focus on racial or ethnic differences runs the risk of undervaluing the great diversity that exists among persons within groups. However, this risk needs to be weighed against the fact that in epidemiologic and clinical research, racial and ethnic categories are useful for generating and exploring hypotheses about environmental and genetic risk factors, as well as interactions between risk factors, for important medical outcomes. Erecting barriers to the collection of information such as race and ethnic background may provide protection against the aforementioned risks; however, it will simultaneously retard progress in biomedical research and limit the effectiveness of clinical decision making.

RACE AND ETHNIC BACKGROUND AS GEOGRAPHIC AND SOCIOCULTURAL CONSTRUCTS WITH BIOLOGIC RAMIFICATIONS

Definitions of race and ethnic background have often been applied inconsistently.[4] The classification scheme used in the 2000 U.S. Census, which is often

35

used in biomedical research, includes five major groups: black or African American, white, Asian, native Hawaiian or other Pacific Islander, and American Indian or Alaska native. In general, this classification scheme emphasizes the geographic region of origin of a person's ancestry.[5] Ethnic background is a broader construct that takes into consideration cultural tradition, common history, religion, and often a shared genetic heritage.

From the perspective of genetics, structure in the human population is determined by patterns of mating and reproduction. Historically, the greatest force influencing genetic differentiation among humans has been geography. Great physical distances and geographic barriers (e.g., high mountains, large deserts, and large bodies of water) have imposed impediments to human communication and interaction and have led to geographically determined endogamous (i.e., within-group) mating patterns resulting in a genetic substructure that largely follows geographic lines. The past two decades of research in population genetics has also shown that the greatest genetic differentiation in the human population occurs between continentally separated groups.

Endogamous mating within continents has given rise to further subdivisions, often corresponding to ethnic groups. This subdivision is again partially attributable to geography but is also associated with social factors, including religion, culture, language, and other sources of group identification. Thus, ethnic groups are genetically differentiated to varying degrees, depending on the extent of reproductive isolation and endogamy, but typically less so than are continentally defined groups.

Considerable debate has focused on whether race and ethnic identity are primarily social or biologic constructs.[6] Unlike a biologic category such as sex, racial and ethnic categories arose primarily through geographic, social, and cultural forces and, as such, are not stagnant, but potentially fluid. Even though these forces are not biologic in nature, racial or ethnic groups do differ from each other genetically, which has biologic implications.

SOCIOCULTURAL CORRELATES
OF RACE AND ETHNIC BACKGROUND

The racial or ethnic groups described above do not differ from each other solely in terms of genetic makeup, especially in a multiracial and multicultural society such as the United States. Socioeconomic status is strongly correlated with race and ethnic background and is a robust predictor of access to and quality of health care and education, which, in turn, may be associated with differences in the incidence of diseases and the outcomes of those diseases.[7] For example, black Americans with end-stage renal disease are referred for renal transplantation at lower rates than white Americans.[8] Black Americans are also referred for cardiac catheterization less frequently than white Americans.[9] In some cases, these differences may be due to bias on the part of physicians and discriminatory practices in medicine.[10] Nonetheless, racial or ethnic differences in the outcomes of disease sometimes persist even when discrepancies in the use of interventions known to be beneficial are considered. For example, the rate of complications from type 2 diabetes mellitus varies according to racial or ethnic category among members of the same health maintenance organization, despite uniform utilization of outpatient services and after adjustment for levels of education and income, health behavior, and clinical characteristics.[11] The evaluation of whether genetic (as well as nongenetic) differences underlie racial disparities is appropriate in cases in which important racial and ethnic differences persist after socioeconomic status and access to care are properly taken into account.

EVIDENCE OF GENETIC DIFFERENTIATION AMONG RACES

There are estimated to be at least 15 million genetic polymorphisms,[12] and an as yet undefined subgroup of these polymorphisms underlie variation in normal and disease traits. The importance of such variation is underscored by the fact that a change of only a single base pair is required to cause many well-known inherited diseases, such as sickle cell disease, or to increase the risk of common disorders, such as Alzheimer's disease. Studies in population genetics have revealed great genetic variation within racial or ethnic subpopulations, but also substantial variation among the five major racial groups, as defined above.[5] This variation has been demonstrated in at least three ways.

First, investigators studying the population genetics of indigenous groups from around the world have constructed ancestral-tree diagrams showing branching relationships among the various indigenous groups. Despite differences in the types of markers used, these studies have been consistent in showing that the human population has major branches corresponding to the major racial groups, with subbranches within each racial group associated with indigenous groups.[13-15]

Second, analysis of genetic clusters has been applied to persons of diverse ancestry, with a focus on genotypes at multiple genetic loci. These analyses have also consistently resulted in the delineation of major genetic clusters that are associated with racial categories.[16-19] The primary difference between the results of these studies and the categories used by the U.S. Census is that South, Central, and West Asians cluster with Europeans and are separate from East Asians.

Third, studies have examined the distribution of differences among racial groups in the frequency of alleles (genetic variants) at both microsatellite and single-nucleotide-polymorphism (SNP) markers, demonstrating a median difference in allele frequency of 15 to 20 percent, with 10 percent of markers showing a difference of 40 percent or more.[5, 20, 21] Thus, for an allele with a frequency of 20 percent or greater in one racial group, the odds are in favor of seeing the same variant in another racial group. However, variants with a frequency below that level are more likely to be race-specific. This race-specificity of variants is particularly common among Africans, who display greater genetic variability than other racial groups and have a larger number of low-frequency alleles.[17] These results indicate that the frequency of variant alleles underlying disease or normal phenotypes can vary substantially among racial groups, leading to differences in the frequency of the phenotypes themselves. Such differences in frequency are also found among ethnic groups, but these differences are typically not as great. Furthermore, self-defined ancestry is very highly correlated with genetically defined clusters.[5, 19]

GENETIC DIFFERENCES IN DISEASE AMONG RACIAL AND ETHNIC GROUPS

To what degree does genetic variability account for medically important differences in disease outcomes among racial and ethnic groups? The answer depends on the frequency of the genetic variants or alleles (mutations) underlying the susceptibility to the disease. For mendelian disorders, the relevance of race and ethnic background is readily apparent. Mutations that have frequencies of less than 2 percent are nearly always race-specific and, in fact, are often specific to single ethnic groups within a given race. For example, numerous mutations with frequencies in this range occur uniquely in Ashkenazi Jews, French Canadians, the Amish, or European gypsies. This is because such populations descend from a relatively small number of founders and have remained endogamous for a large part of their history. Mutant alleles with frequencies of more than 2 percent but less than 20 percent are typically prevalent within single racial groups but not in other racial groups. For example, hemochromatosis is associated with a mutant allele (C282Y) found in all European groups and at especially high frequency (8 to 10 percent) in northern Europeans, but is virtually absent in nonwhite groups.[22]

"Complex" genetic disorders such as asthma, cancer, diabetes, and atherosclerosis are most likely due to multiple, potentially interacting, genes and environmental factors and are thus more challenging to study. The genetic determinants of the majority of these disorders are currently poorly understood, but the few examples that do exist demonstrate clinically important racial and ethnic differences in gene frequency. For example, factor V Leiden, a genetic variant that confers an increased risk of venous thromboembolic disease, is present in about 5 percent of white people. In contrast, this variant is rarely found in East Asians and Africans (prevalence, $\leq$1 percent).[23, 24] Susceptibility to Crohn's disease is associated with three polymorphic genetic variants in the *CARD15* gene in whites[25]; none of these genetic variants were found in Japanese patients with Crohn's disease.[26] Another important gene that affects a complex trait is *CCR5*—a receptor used by the human immunodeficiency virus (HIV) to enter cells. As many as 25 percent of white people (especially in northern Europe) are heterozygous for the *CCR5–delta32* variant, which is protective against HIV infection and progression, whereas this variant is virtually absent in other groups, thus suggesting racial and ethnic differences in protection against HIV.[27]

Other alleles occur in all ethnic groups but with highly variable frequency. Increasingly, researchers and clinicians are focusing on identifying and studying the genetic variants that influence responses to drugs and the metabolism of drugs (an area of study termed pharmacogenetics). One example is *N*-acetyltransferase 2 (NAT2), an enzyme involved in the detoxification of many carcinogens and the metabolism of many commonly used drugs. Genetic variants of NAT2 result in two phenotypes, slow and rapid acetylators. Population-based studies of NAT2 and its metabolites have shown that the slow-acetylator phenotype ranges in frequency from approximately 14 percent among East Asians to 34 percent among black Americans to 54 percent among whites.[28] Genetic variants of NAT2 are important because they may predict toxic effects of drugs and because they may contribute to racial and ethnic variation in the incidence of environmentally induced cancers.

RACIAL AND ETHNIC DIFFERENCES AS CLUES TO INTERACTIONS

Even when all racial and ethnic groups share a genetic variant that causes a disease, studies of different groups may offer important insights. One of the best-known examples of a gene that affects a complex disease is APOE. A patient harboring a variant of this gene, *APOE* ε4, has a substantially increased risk of Alzheimer's disease. *APOE* ε4 is relatively common and is seen in all racial and ethnic groups, albeit at different frequencies, ranging from 9 percent in Japanese populations to 14 percent in white populations to 19 percent in black American populations.[29] However, a recent meta-analysis has demonstrated that the effect of *APOE* ε4 on the risk of Alzheimer's disease varies according to race.[29] Homozygosity for the ε4 allele increases risk by a factor of 33 in Japanese populations and by a factor of 15 in white populations, but only by a factor of 6 in black American populations; similarly, heterozygosity for the ε4 allele increases the risk by a factor of 5.6 in Japanese populations, by a factor of 3.0 in white populations, and by a factor of 1.1 in black American populations. Although the reason for this variation in risk remains unknown, it suggests that there may be genetic or environmental modifiers of this gene. Thus, even when a genetic determinant of a complex disease is present in all racial and ethnic groups, racial and ethnic classification may offer additional important insights.

RACIALLY ADMIXED POPULATIONS

Although studies of population genetics have clustered persons into a small number of groups corresponding roughly to five major racial categories, such classification is not completely discontinuous, because there has been intermixing among groups both over the course of history and in recent times. In particular, genetic admixture, or the presence in a population of persons with multiple races or ethnic backgrounds, is well documented in the border regions of continents and may represent genetic gradations (clines)—for example, among East Africans (e.g., Ethiopians)[18] and some central Asian groups.[19] In the United States, mixture among different racial groups has occurred recently, although in the 2000 U.S. Census, the majority of respondents still identified themselves as members of a single racial group. Genetic studies of black Americans have documented a range of 7 to 20 percent white admixture, depending on the geographic location of the population studied.[30] Despite the admixture, black Americans, as a group, are still genetically similar to Africans. Hispanics, the largest and fastest growing minority population in the United States, are an admixed group that includes white and Native American ancestry, as well as African ancestry.[31] The proportions of admixture in this group also vary according to geographic region.

Although the categorization of admixed groups poses special challenges, groups containing persons with varying levels of admixture can also be particularly useful for genetic-epidemiologic studies. For example, Williams et al. studied the association between the degree of white admixture and the incidence of type 2 diabetes mellitus among Pima Indians.[32] They found that the self-reported degree of white admixture (reported as a percentage) was strongly correlated with protection from diabetes in this population. Furthermore, as noted above, information on race or ethnic background can provide important clues to effects of culture, access to care, and bias on the part of caregivers, even in genetically admixed populations. It is also important to recognize that many groups (e.g., most Asian groups) are highly underrepresented both in the population of the United States and in typical surveys of population genetics, relative to their global numbers. Thus, primary categories that are relevant for the current U.S. population might not be optimal for a globally derived sample.

RISKS ENTAILED BY IGNORING RACE IN BIOMEDICAL RESEARCH AND CLINICAL PRACTICE

Given its controversial social and political history, it may be tempting to abandon the notion of race altogether, particularly if we believe that continued attention to differences among races may perpetuate discrepancies in health status and well-being. Indeed, some have advocated discontinuing the collection of information about race and ethnic background, presumably as a way of protecting minority groups. In California, advocates of this move are pushing for a state law—through the Racial Privacy Initiative[33]—that would prohibit racial classification by the state or other public entities. Although this initiative formally excludes a ban on classification for the purposes of medical research, the abolition of the collection of data on race or ethnic group for all other purposes would eliminate these data from many public data bases on which clinicians and scientists rely in order to make meaningful inferences about the effects of race and ethnic background on health and disease in persons and populations.

We believe that ignoring race and ethnic background would be detrimental to the very populations and persons that this approach allegedly seeks to protect. Information about patients' ethnic or racial group is imperative for the identification, tracking, and investigation of the reasons for racial and ethnic differences in the prevalence and severity of disease and in responses to treatment. This information is also crucial for identifying different risk-factor profiles even when a disease does not occur with dramatically different frequencies in different racial or ethnic groups. Furthermore, knowledge of a person's ancestry may facilitate testing, diagnosis, and treatment when genetic factors are involved. For example, there are already tests to screen for disease-causing mutations that are tailored to specific racial or ethnic groups. Currently, racial and ethnic minorities in the United States are underrepresented in many clinical studies.[34] If investigators ignored race and ethnic background in research studies and persons were sampled randomly, the overwhelming majority of participants in clinical studies in the United States would be white, and minority populations would never be adequately sampled.[5] In cases in which there are important racial and ethnic differences in the causes of disease or other outcomes or in which there are interactions between race or ethnic background and other factors contributing to these outcomes, such patterns would never be discovered, their causes could not be identified, and the appropriate interventions would never be applied in the groups in which they were needed. Despite the fact that the National Institutes of Health requires reporting of all racial or ethnic groups participating in biomedical research, limited progress has been made in the inclusion of minority groups.

CONCLUSIONS

There are racial and ethnic differences in the causes, expression, and prevalence of various diseases. The relative importance of bias, culture, socioeconomic status, access to care, and environmental and genetic influences on the development of disease is an empirical question that, in most cases, remains unanswered. Although there are potential social costs associated with linking race or ethnic background with genetics[35], we believe that these potential costs are outweighed by the benefits in terms of diagnosis and research. Ignoring racial and ethnic differences in medicine and biomedical research will not make them disappear. Rather than ignoring these differences, scientists should continue to use them as starting points for further research. Only by focusing attention on these issues can we hope to understand better the variations among racial and ethnic groups in the prevalence and severity of diseases and in responses to treatment. Such understanding provides the opportunity to develop strategies for the improvement of health outcomes for everyone.

From the Lung Biology Center (E.G.B., N.C., D.S.), the Division of General Internal Medicine (E.Z., E.J.P.-S.), the Department of Medicine (E.G.B., E.Z., N.C., E.J.P.-S., D.S.), and the Medical Effectiveness Research Center for Diverse Populations (E.G.B., E.Z., EJ.P.-S.), University of California, San Francisco; and San Francisco General Hospital (E.G.B., N.C., D.S.)—both in San Francisco; the Division of Epidemiology, Department of Health Research and Policy (S.L.G.), and the Department of Genetics (N.R.), Stanford University School of Medicine, and the Department of Statistics (H.T) and the Department of Anthropological Sciences (J.L.M.), Stanford University—both in Stanford, Calif.; the Northern California Cancer Center, Union City, Calif. (S.L.G.); and the Department of Epidemiology and Health Services Research, Division of Research, Kaiser Permanente, Oakland, Calif. (AJ.K., N.R.). Address reprint requests to Dr. González Burchard at the University of California, San Francisco, San Francisco, CA 94143–0833, or at eburch@ itsa.ucsf.edu.

Drs. González Burchard and Ziv contributed equally to the chapter.

NOTES

1. Lander E. Cracking the code of life. Boston: WGBH, 2001(transcript).
2. Angier N. Do races differ? Not really, genes show. New York Times. August 22, 2000:Fl.
3. Schwartz RS. Racial profiling in medical research. N Engl J Med 2001; 344:1392–3.
4. Sankar P, Cho MK. Genetics: toward a new vocabulary of human genetic variation. Science 2002;298:1337–8.
5. Risch N, Burchard E, Ziv E, Tang H. Categorization of humans in biomedical research: genes, race and disease. Genome Biol 2002; 3(7):comment 2007. 1–comment 2007.12.
6. Kaufinan JS, Cooper RS. Considerations for use of racial/ethnic classification in etiologic research. Am J Epidemiol 2001;154:291–8.
7. Smedley BD, Stith AY, Nelson AR, eds. Unequal treatment: confronting race and ethnic disparities in health care. Washington, D.C.: National Academy Press, 2002.
8. Epstein AM, Ayanian JZ, Keogh JH, et al. Racial disparities in access to renal transplantation: clinically appropriate or due to underuse or overuse? N Engl J Med 2000;343:1537–44.
9. Peterson ED, Wright SM, Daley J, Thibault GE. Racial variation in cardiac procedure use and survival following acute myocardial infarction in the Department of Veterans Affairs. JAMA 1994;271: 1175–80.
10. Schulman KA, Berlin JA, Harless W, et al. The effect of race and sex on physicians' recommendations for cardiac catheterization. N Engl J Med 1999;340:618–26. [Erratum, N Engl J Med 1999;340: 1130.]
11. Karter AJ, Ferrara A, Liu JY, Moffet HH, Ackerson LM, Selby JV. Ethnic disparities in diabetic complications in an insured population. JAMA 2002;287:2519–27.
12. Judson P, Salisbury B, Schneider J, Windemuth A, Stephens JC. How many SNPs does a genome-wide haplotype map require? Pharmacogenomics 2002;3:379–91.
13. Calafell F, Shuster A, Speed WC, Kidd JR, Kidd KK. Short tandem repeat polymorphism evolution in humans. Eur J Hum Genet 1998;6:38–49.
14. Bowcock AM, Ruiz-Linares A, Tomfohrde J, Minch E, Kidd JR, Cavalli-Sforza LL. High resolution of human evolutionary trees with polymorphic microsatellites. Nature 1994;368:455–7.
15. Bowcock AM, Kidd JR, Mountain JL, et al. Drift, admixture, and selection in human evolution: a study with DNA polymorphisms. Proc Natl Acad Sci U S A 1991;88:839–43.
16. Mountain JL, Cavalli-Sforza LL. Multilocus genotypes, a tree of individuals, and human evolutionary history. Am J Hum Genet 1997;61:705–18.
17. Stephens JC, Schneider JA, Tanguay DA, et al. Haplotype variation and linkage disequilibrium in 313 human genes. Science 2001; 293:489–93. [Erratum, Science 2001;293:1048.]
18. Wilson JF, Weale ME, Smith AC, et al. Population genetic structure of variable drug response. Nat Genet 2001;29:265–9.

19. Rosenberg NA, Pritchard JK, Weber JL, et al. Genetic structure of human populations. Science 2002;298:2381–5.

20. Dean M, Stephens JC, Winkler C, et al. Polymorphic admixture typing in human ethnic populations. Am J Hum Genet 1994;55: 788–808.

21. Smith MW, Lautenberger JA, Shin HD, et al. Markers for mapping by admixture linkage disequilibrium in African American and Hispanic populations. Am J Hum Genet 2001;69:1080–94.

22. Merryweather-Clarke AT, Pointon JJ, Jouanolle AM, Rochette J, Robson KJ. Geography of HFE C282Y and H63D mutations. Genet Test 2000;4:183–98.

23. Ridker PM, Miletich JP, Hennekens CH, Buring JE. Ethnic distribution of factor V Leiden in 4047 men and women—implications for venous thromboembolism screening. JAMA 1997;277:1305–7.

24. Shen MC, Lin JS, Tsay W. High prevalence of antithrombin III, protein C and protein S deficiency, but no factor V Leiden mutation in venous thrombophilic Chinese patients in Taiwan. Thromb Res 1997;87:377–85.

25. Hugot JP, Chamaillard M, Zouali H, et al. Association of NOD2 leucin-rich repeat variants with susceptibility to Crohn's disease. Nature 2001;411:599–603.

26. Yamazaki K, Takazoe M, Tanaka T, Kazumori T, Nakamura Y. Absence of mutation in the NOD2/CARD15 gene among 483 Japanese patients with Crohn's disease. J Hum Genet 2002;47:469–72.

27. Stephens JC, Reich DE, Goldstein DB, et al. Dating the origin of the CCR5–Delta32 AIDS-resistance allele by the coalescence of haplotypes. Am J Hum Gen 1998;62:1507–15.

28. Yu MC, Skipper PL, Taghizadeh K, et al. Acetylator phenotype, aminobiphenyl-hemoglobin adduct levels, and bladder cancer risk in white, black, and Asian men in Los Angeles, California. J Natl Cancer Inst 1994;86:712–6.

29. Farrer LA, Cupples LA, Haines JL, et al. Effects of age, sex, and ethnicity on the association between apolipoprotein E genotype and Alzheimer disease: a meta-analysis. JAMA 1997;278:1349–56.

30. Parra EJ, Marcini A, Akey J, et al. Estimatng African American admixture proportions by use of population-specific alleles. Am J Hum Genet 1998;63:1839–51.

31. Hanis CL, Hewett-Emmett D, Bertin TK, Schull WJ. Origins of U.S. Hispanics: implications for diabetes. Diabetes Care 1991;14: 618–27.

32. Williams RC, Long JC, Hanson RL, Sievers ML, Knowler WC. Individual estimates of European genetic admixture associated with lower body-mass index, plasma glucose, and prevalence of type 2 diabetes in Pima Indians. Am J Hum Genet 2000;66:527–38.

33. Racial privacy initiative. Sacramento, Calif.: American Civil Rights Coalition, 2002. (Accessed February 28, 2003, at http://www. racialprivacy.org.)

34. Gifford AL, Cunningham WE, Heslin KC, et al. Participation in research and access to experimental treatments by HIV-infected patients. N Engl J Med 2002;346:1373–82.

35. Foster MW, Sharp RR. Race, ethnicity, and genomics: social classifications as proxies of biological heterogeneity. Genome Res 2002;12:844–50.

4

The Model State Emergency Health Powers Act: Planning for and Response to Bioterrorism and Naturally Occurring Infectious Diseases

*Lawrence O. Gostin, Jason W. Sapsin, Stephen P. Teret,
Scott Burris, Julie Samia Mair, James G. Hodge, Jr.,
and Jon S. Vernick*

The Center for Law and the Public's Health at Georgetown and Johns Hopkins Universities drafted the Model State Emergency Health Powers Act (MSEHPA or Model Act) at the request of the Centers for Disease Control and Prevention. The Model Act provides state actors with the powers they need to detect and contain bioterrorism or a naturally occurring disease outbreak. Legislative bills based on the MSEHPA have been introduced in 34 states. Problems of obsolescence, inconsistency, and inadequacy may render current state laws ineffective or even counterproductive. State laws often date back to the early 20th century and have been built up in layers over the years. They frequently predate the vast changes in the public health sciences and constitutional law.

The Model Act is structured to reflect 5 basic public health functions to be facilitated by law: (1) *preparedness,* comprehensive planning for a public health emergency; (2) *surveillance,* measures to detect and track public health emergencies; (3) *management of property,* ensuring adequate availability of vaccines, pharmaceuticals, and hospitals, as well as providing power to abate hazards to the public's health; (4) *protection of persons,* powers to compel vaccination, testing, treatment, isolation, and quarantine when clearly necessary; and (5) *communication,* providing clear and authoritative information to the public. The Model Act also contains a modernized, extensive set of principles and requirements to safeguard personal rights. Law can be a tool to improve public health preparedness. A constitutional democracy must balance the common good with respect for personal dignity, toleration of groups, and adherence to principles of justice.

Safeguarding the public's health, safety, and security took on new meaning and urgency after the attacks on the World Trade Center in New York City and the Pentagon in Arlington, Va, on September 11, 2001. On October 4, 2001, a Florida man was diagnosed with inhalational anthrax.[1, 2] The intentional dispersal of anthrax through the US postal system in New York, Washington, and other locations resulted in 5 confirmed deaths, hundreds of persons treated, and thousands tested.[3] The potential for new, larger, and more sophisticated attacks has created a sense of vulnerability. National attention has urgently turned to the need to rapidly detect and react to bioterrorism, as well as to naturally occurring infectious diseases.

In the aftermath of September 11, the president and the Congress began a process to strengthen the public health infrastructure.[4] The Center for Law and the Public's Health at Georgetown and Johns Hopkins Universities drafted the Model State Emergency Health Powers Act (MSEHFA or the Model Act[5] at the request of the Centers for Disease Control and Prevention (CDC) and in collaboration with members of national organizations representing governors, legislators, attorneys general, and health commissioners. Because the power to act to preserve the public's health is constitutionally reserved primarily to the states as an exercise of their police powers,[6] the Model Act is designed for state, not federal, legislative consideration. It provides the responsible state actors with the powers they need to detect and contain a potentially catastrophic disease outbreak and, at the same time, protect individual rights and freedoms. Legislative bills based on the MSEHPA have been introduced in 34 states and the District of Columbia; 16 states and the District of Columbia already have enacted a version of the act (as of June 26, 2002, states enacting or expected shortly to enact legislation influenced by the Model Act were Arizona, Florida, Georgia, Hawaii, Maine, Maryland, Minnesota, Missouri, New Hampshire, New Mexico, Oklahoma, South Carolina, South Dakota, Tennessee, Utah, and Virginia).[7, 8] This article explains the need for law reform, describes the main provisions of the Model Act, and discusses the delicate balance between public health and civil liberties in a constitutional democracy.

BACKGROUND

Both naturally occurring infectious diseases and deliberate acts of bioterrorism pose threats to public health. Historically, major infectious disease outbreaks have killed far more people than war: approximately 25 million Europeans, over a quarter of the population, died of bubonic plague in the 14th century[9]; diseases such as smallpox, measles, influenza, typhus, and bubonic plague killed an estimated 95% of pre-Columbian Native American populations[10];

and a worldwide influenza epidemic in 1918–1919 resulted in the death of 21 million people.[11] While infectious disease may no longer be the leading cause of death in the United States because of advancements in hygiene, nutrition, and medicine, the death toll is still substantial.[12] Each year approximately 170,000 people in the United States die from infectious diseases.[13]

Preventing major disease outbreaks poses as great a challenge as ever before. The globalization of travel and trade allows for the widespread, rapid transmission of disease. A person infected in Hong Kong can travel to the United States in less than a day. Large concentrations of people also facilitate the spread of disease, and many cities have populations in the millions. Even in contemporary societies human populations remain in close proximity to animal populations. Some of the most deadly human diseases are believed to have evolved from animal diseases.[10]

In addition to the threat of severe naturally occurring diseases, both recent events and several reports highlight the threat of bioterrorism. We define *bioterrorism* as the intentional use of a pathogen or biological product to cause harm to a human, animal, plant, or other living organism to influence the conduct of government or to intimidate or coerce a civilian population. A report by the National Intelligence Council for the Central Intelligence Agency concluded that infectious disease is not only a public health issue but also a problem of national security: the US population is vulnerable to bioterrorism as well as emerging and reemerging infectious diseases.[13] In 1998, the US Commission on National Security in the 21st Century concluded that biological agents are the most likely choice of weapons for disaffected states and groups. Biological weapons are nearly as easy to develop, far more lethal, and will likely become easier to deliver than chemical weapons and, unlike nuclear weapons, biological weapons are inexpensive to produce and the risk of detection is low.[14] In 1993, the US Congressional Office of Technology Assessment estimated that the aerosolized release of 100 kg of anthrax spores upwind of Washington, DC, could result in approximately 130,000 to 3 million deaths, a weapon as deadly as a hydrogen bomb.[15]

For years, experts have been calling attention to the threat of bioterrorism and the unique problems that arise in modern society.[16–20] The Internet allows for the widespread dissemination of information on biological agents and technology. Advancements in biotechnology make bioproduction capabilities accessible to individuals with limited experience. The dual-use nature of this knowledge and technology, allowing for both legitimate and illicit use, makes tracking and identifying bioterrorists much more difficult. And while certain countries are known or suspected to have biological weapons programs, non-state actors have become important as well.[14] Documents recovered in

Afghanistan suggest that Al Qaeda has conducted extensive research on weapons that can cause mass fatalities, including biological weapons.[21]

Government and public health officials must be able to react quickly and intelligently to a potentially catastrophic disease outbreak, whether intentionally instigated or naturally occurring. Two exercises, Dark Winter (smallpox)[22] and TOPOFF (plague),[23] simulated biological attacks in the United States to test government response and raise awareness of the bioterrorism threat. Both simulations demonstrated serious weaknesses in the US public health system that could prevent an effective response to bioterrorism or severe naturally occurring infectious diseases.[14–25]

THE NEED FOR LAW REFORM

Law has long been considered an important tool of public health.[26] While federal law-making authority is constitutionally limited in scope, as an exercise of their broader police powers, states have more flexibility in legislating to protect the public's health. State public health laws create a mission for public health authorities, assign their functions, and specify the manner in which they may exercise their authority.[27] Prior to September 11, 2001, some states had legislatively (eg, Colorado[28]) or administratively (eg, Rhode Island[29]) developed public health response plans for a bioterrorism event. However, problems of obsolescence, inconsistency, and inadequacy may render some public health laws ineffective or even counterproductive.[30] Reforming state public health law can improve the legal infrastructure to help respond to bioterrorism and other emerging threats.

State public health statutes frequently are outdated and were built up in layers during the 20th century in response to each new disease threat. Consequently, these laws often do not reflect contemporary scientific understandings of disease (eg, surveillance, prevention, and response) or legal norms for protection of individual rights. When many of these statutes were written, public health sciences, such as epidemiology and biostatistics, were in their infancy and, modern prevention and treatment methods did not exist.

At the same time, many existing public health laws pre-date the vast changes in constitutional (eg, equal protection and due process) and statutory (eg, disability discrimination) law that have transformed social and legal conceptions of individual rights. Failure to reform these laws may leave public health authorities vulnerable to legal challenge on grounds that they are unconstitutional or preempted by modern federal statutes. Even if state public health law is not challenged in court, public health authorities may feel unsure about applying old legal remedies to modern health threats. The Minnesota state legislature has recently passed a bill that, like the Model Act, permits quarantine and isolation in limited circumstances but makes these practices subject to modernized, significant personal safeguards including due process.[31]

Health codes among the 50 states and territories have evolved independently, leading to profound variation in the structure, substance, and procedures for detecting, controlling, and preventing disease. Ordinarily different state approaches are not a problem, but variation could prevent or delay an efficient response in a multistate public health emergency. Infectious diseases are rarely confined to single jurisdictions but pose risks within whole regions or the nation itself. Coordination among state and national authorities is vital but is undermined by disparate legal structures.

Public health laws remain fragmented within states as well as among them. Most state statutes have evolved over time so that, even within the same state, different rules may apply depending on the particular disease in question. This means that necessary authority (eg, screening, reporting, or compulsory treatment) may be absent for a given disease. For example, when a resurgence of multidrug resistant tuberculosis swept major metropolitan areas in the 1990s, many statutes did not allow for directly observed therapy.[32] Worse still, state laws can be so complex that they may not be well understood by health practitioners or their attorneys. Laws that are ambiguous prevent agencies from acting rapidly and decisively in an emergency. Many current laws not only provide insufficient authority to act but might actually thwart effective action. This is evident when one examines the key variables for public health preparedness: planning, coordination and communication, surveillance, management of property, and protection of persons.

State statutes generally fail to require planning or to establish mechanisms. As a result, most states have not systematically designed a strategy to respond to public health emergencies. Perhaps the most important aspects of planning are clear communication and coordination among responsible governmental officials and the private sector. As the recent anthrax outbreaks demonstrate[33], there should be a defined role for public health, law enforcement, and emergency management agencies. Also, there should be coordination among the various levels (eg, federal, tribal, state, and local) and branches (legislative, executive, and judicial) of government as well as with private actors, particularly the health care and pharmaceutical sectors. Communication and coordination are improved by a systematic planning process that involves all stakeholders. The law can require such planning and sharing of information. However, many public health statutes do not facilitate communication and, due to federal and state privacy concerns, may actually proscribe exchange of vital information among public health, law enforcement, and emergency management agencies. Indeed, some statutes even prohibit sharing data with public health officials in adjoining states by strictly limiting disclosures by the public health agency that holds the data, often in the interest of protecting individual privacy.[34] Laws that complicate or hinder data communication among states and responsible agencies would impede a thorough investigation and response to such a public health emergency.

Surveillance is critical to public health preparedness. Unlike most forms of terrorism, the dispersal of pathogens may not be evident. Early detection could save many lives by triggering an effective containment strategy such as vaccination, treatment, and, if necessary, isolation or quarantine. However, current statutes do not facilitate surveillance and may even prevent monitoring. For example, many states do not require timely reporting for certain dangerous (Category A) agents of bioterrorism such as smallpox, anthrax, plague, botulism, tularemia, and viral hemorrhagic fevers.[35] In fact, virtually no state requires immediate reporting for all the critical agents identified by the CDC.[36] At the same time, states do not require, and may actually prohibit, public health agencies from monitoring data collected in the health care system. Private information held by hospitals, managed care organizations, and pharmacies that might lead to early detection (eg, unusual clusters of fevers or gastrointestinal symptoms) may be unavailable to public health officials.[32] New federal health information privacy protections may unintentionally impede the flow of data from private to public sectors despite regulators' attempt to broadly exempt public health information sharing from nondisclosure rules.[37]

Coercive powers are the most controversial aspects of any legal system. Nevertheless, they may be necessary to manage property or protect persons in a public health emergency. There are numerous circumstances that might require management of property in a public health emergency (eg, shortages of vaccines, medicines, hospital beds, or facilities for disposal of corpses). It may even be necessary to close facilities or destroy property that is contaminated or dangerous. Even in the case of a relatively small outbreak, such as the recent anthrax attacks, the government considered the need to compulsorily license proprietary medications and destroy contaminated facilities.[6] The law must provide authority, with fair safeguards, to manage property that is needed to contain a serious health threat.

There similarly may be a need to exercise powers over individuals to avert a significant threat to the public's health. Vaccination, testing, physical examination, treatment, isolation, and quarantine each may help contain the spread of infectious diseases. Although the vast majority of people probably will comply willingly (because it is in their interests and/or desirable for the common welfare), some compulsory powers are necessary for those who will not comply. Provided those powers are bounded by legal safeguards, individuals should be required to yield some of their autonomy, liberty, or property to protect the health and security of the community.

THE MODEL STATE EMERGENCY HEALTH POWERS ACT

From a practical and political perspective, it is important that any model law draw its legitimacy from recognized sources of authority. The MSEHPN's theoretical foundations and structures are derived from existing federal or state law that offers model language; lessons derived from theoretical exercises such as TOPOFF and Dark Winter; and a meeting of high-level experts in public health, emergency management, and national security, which took place at the Cantigny Conference Center in April 2001.[38] The Center for Law and the Public's Health received comments on the Model Act from government agencies, national organizations, academic institutions, practitioners, and the general public. The Model Act, therefore, expresses an attempted best synthesis of advice, recommendations, and dialogue regarding the purpose of emergency public health law, its proper reach, and the protection of civil liberties and private property (Table 4.1).

Table 4.1 Table of Contents for the Model Act

continued

Table 4.1 Table of Contents for the Model Act (*continued*)

The purpose of the MSEHPA is to facilitate the detection, management, and containment of public health emergencies while appropriately safeguarding personal and proprietary interests. The Model Act gives rise to 2 kinds of public health powers and duties: those that exist in the preemergency environment (predeclaration powers found in Articles II and III) and a separate group of powers and duties that come into effect only after a state's governor declares a public health emergency (the postdeclaration powers of Articles V, VI, and VII). Postdeclaration powers deliberately are broader and more robust.

Under Article IV, a governor may declare a public health emergency only if a series of demanding threshold conditions are met: (1) an occurrence or imminent threat of an illness or health condition, that (2) is caused by bioterrorism or a new or reemerging infectious agent or biological toxin previously controlled and that (3) also poses a high probability of a large number of deaths, a large number of serious or long-term disabilities, or widespread exposure to an infectious or toxic agent that poses a significant risk of substantial future harm to a large number of persons. Recognizing the continuing threat of infectious disease, the Model Act as drafted is not limited to bioterrorism emergencies; a mass epidemic could be sufficiently severe to trigger the Model Act's provisions even if naturally occurring. States may therefore choose to enhance and further strengthen the threshold conditions for invoking the Model Act, perhaps by including a requirement that the security, safety, or normal operation of the state be threatened before an emergency may be declared. States may also choose an all-hazards approach that adds chemical and nuclear threats to the biological threats contemplated by the Model Act. The MSEHPA requires the governor to consult with the public health authority and other experts prior to declaring an emergency (unless the delay would endanger the public's health), specifies minimum information to be provided in an emergency declaration, and authorizes the suspension of ordinary state rules or regulations to facilitate emergency response. The legislature, by majority vote, may discontinue the state of emergency at any time.

The predeclaration powers and duties are those necessary to prepare for and promptly identify a public health emergency. Under Article II (Planning for a Public Health Emergency), the Public Health Emergency Planning Commission (appointed by the governor) must prepare a plan which includes coordination of services; procurement of necessary materials and supplies; housing, feeding, and caring for affected populations (with appropriate regard for their physical and cultural/social needs); and the proper vaccination and treatment of individuals in the event of a public health emergency.

Article III (Measures to Detect and Track Public Health Emergencies) addresses measures necessary to detect initially and then to follow a developing public health emergency, including prompt (24 hours) reporting requirements for health care providers, pharmacists, veterinarians, and laboratories. Public health professionals must interview and counsel persons exposed to illnesses, which may cause a public health emergency, and their contacts. Additionally, the public health authority must investigate physical materials or facilities endangering the public's health. The Model Act recognizes that exchange of relevant data among lead agencies is essential to assure the public's health and security. Therefore, public health, emergency management, and public safety authorities are required to share information necessary to prevent, treat, control, or investigate a public health emergency.

The Model Act provides "special powers" that may be used only after a governor declares a state of public health emergency. Article V (Management of Property) provides that the state's designated public health authority may close, decontaminate, or procure facilities and materials to respond to a public health emergency, safely dispose of infectious waste, and obtain and deploy health care supplies. The authorities are required to exercise their powers with respect for cultural and religious beliefs and practices such as observing, wherever possible, religious laws regarding burial. Compensation of private property owners is provided if there is a *taking* (ie, the government confiscates private property for public purposes, such as the use of a private infirmary to treat and/or isolate patients). No compensation would be provided for a *nuisance abatement* (ie, the government destroys property or closes an establishment that poses a serious health threat). This comports with the extant constitutional takings jurisprudence of the Supreme Court.[39] If the government were forced to compensate for all nuisance abatements, it would significantly chill public health regulation.

The provisions for protection of persons found in Article VI (Protection of Persons) deal with some of the most sensitive areas within the MSEHPA. The Model Act permits public health authorities to physically examine or test individuals as necessary to diagnose or to treat illness, vaccinate or treat individuals to prevent or ameliorate an infectious disease, and isolate or quarantine individuals to prevent or limit the transmission of a contagious disease. The public health authority also may waive licensing requirements for health care professionals and direct them to assist in vaccination, testing, examination, and treatment of patients.

While the Model Act reaffirms the authority over persons and property that health agencies have always had, it supplements these traditional public health powers with a modernized, extensive set of conditions, principles, and requirements governing the use of personal control measures that are now often lacking in state public health law. Public health officials are explicitly directed to respect individual religious objections to vaccination and treatment. Officials must follow specified legal standards before using isolation or quarantine, which are authorized only to prevent the transmission of contagious disease to others and must be by the least restrictive means available. This allows individuals, for example, to be confined in their own homes. The Model Act also affords explicit protections to persons in isolation or quarantine that go beyond most existing state laws: the public health authority is affirmatively charged with maintaining places of isolation or quarantine in a safe and hygienic manner; regularly monitoring the health of residents; and systematically and competently meeting the needs of persons isolated or quarantined for adequate food, clothing, shelter, means of communication, medication, and medical care. Orders for isolation or quarantine are subject to judicial review, under strict time guidelines, and with appointed counsel; the Model Act also provides for expedited judicial relief.

Finally, the Model Act provides for a set of postdeclaration powers and duties to ensure appropriate public information and communication (Article VII: Public Information Regarding Public Health Emergency). The public health authority must provide information to the public regarding the emergency, including protective measures to be taken and information regarding access to mental health support. Experience following September 11th and the anthrax attacks demonstrated the need for an authoritative spokesperson for public health providing comprehensible and accurate information. These events also revealed the significant mental health implications of terrorism on the population.[40]

The Model Act also recognizes that if government officials, health professionals, and others are to fulfill their responsibilities for preventing and responding to a serious health threat, they should not fear unwarranted liability. Consequently, MSEHPA affords persons exercising authority under the Model Act immunity from liability except for gross negligence or willful misconduct.

Taken as a whole, MSEHPA resolves a series of difficult policy debates in which the public health goals of facilitating the detection, management, and containment of public health emergencies are balanced against the need to safeguard individuals' civil rights, liberties, and property. The Model Act is an outgrowth of a process to identify and legitimize critical public health functions against a framework of personal rights and freedoms protected by law.

CIVIL LIBERTIES AND THE EXERCISE OF EMERGENCY POWERS

The Model Act is designed to be triggered by an extreme public health emergency comparable with the sudden, devastating epidemics of the 19th century. [41, 42] Emergency health powers by definition are a concession to the fact that normal systems of civil governance may break down under the pressure of widespread sudden death or illness, even as the outbreak demands a decisive response. The exercise of emergency powers to control the movement of individuals and populations, and to seize property, poses risks to personal and economic liberties. It is important, however, to consider carefully the nature of these risks as understood since the founding of the Republic.[43] The rights of liberty, due process, and property are fundamental but not absolute. Justice Harlan in the foundational Supreme Court case of *Jacobson v Massachusetts* (1905) wrote: "There are manifold restraints to which every person is necessarily subject for the common good. On any other basis organized society could not exist with safety to its members."[44] Similarly, private property was held subject to the restriction that it not be used in a way that posed a health hazard, as Lemuel Shaw of the Massachusetts Supreme Judicial Court observed in 1851: "We think it settled principle, growing out of the nature of well ordered civil society, that every holder of property . . . holds it under the implied liability that it shall not be injurious to the right of the community."[45] "It is unquestionable," wrote the Maine Supreme Court in 1876, "that the legislature can confer powers upon public officers, for the protection of the public health. . . . The individual right sinks in the necessity to provide for the public good."[46]

These doctrines remain lively today in the United States[6] and under international law.[47] Even in principle, it would be almost disingenuous to argue that individuals whose movements or property pose a significant risk of harm to their communities have a "right" to be free of interference necessary to control the threat, or that property rights trump the protection of the common good from extreme peril. There is simply no basis for this argument in constitutional law and perhaps little more in political philosophy. These observations do not dispose of the serious threats to individual freedoms posed by the exercise of governmental power in a perceived emergency. Rather, they focus attention on what has been the real contention of parties opposing health actions: not the right to be free of any restraint, but the right to be free of a particular restraint that is not justified under the circumstances. It is not improper to restrain the free enjoyment of liberty, privacy, or property per se, but to do so unnecessarily arbitrarily, or brutally. The restraint of liberty, privacy, or property could lack justification in several ways: the problem being addressed does not exist or is not as serious as believed, the measure taken is unresponsive to the problem, or the measure is more intrusive or restrictive than necessary to ameliorate the threat. Due process as afforded under the Model Act is an important means of forestalling or correcting these kinds of errors. It is also right intrinsically even when an emergency measure is justified. Compulsory powers should be carried out in a way that respects personal dignity and tolerates racial, religious, or ethnic differences.

Some commentators criticize the Model Act for including compulsory powers at all, arguing that governors may deliberately misuse their authority.[48] This criticism, however, ignores 3 fundamental elements of the Model Act. First, MSEHPA does not simply establish compulsory powers but creates the conditions for public health preparedness (eg, planning, surveillance, and communication). Second, compulsory power has always been a part of public health law, because it is sometimes necessary to prevent or ameliorate unacceptable threats to the common good. Third, MSEHPA actually affords greater safeguards of civil liberties than exist under traditional infectious disease laws (eg, providing checks and balances against government abuses, clear standards for the exercise of power, and rigorous procedural due process). A civil rights society must reduce the risk of error and provide people with a timely and meaningful opportunity to correct mistakes and be made whole in instances of abuse. A sharper focus on the practical civil liberties issues posed by emergencies suggests 4 principled limitations. Agency actions should be (1) necessary to avert a significant risk, in the first instance in the judgment of health officials and ultimately, with reasonable deference, to the satisfaction of a judge; (2) reasonably well-tailored to address the risk in the sense officials do not overreach or go beyond a necessary and appropriate response; (3) authorized in a manner allowing public scrutiny and oversight; and (4) correctable in the event of an unreasonable mistake. The Model Act was drafted to satisfy each of these criteria. In these respects, MSEHPA is an improvement over many state laws that do not provide standards or procedures for the exercise of power.[28]

Appropriate statutory language, of course, is only part of the solution to the problem of erroneous emergency action. The greatest risk to liberties may be that safeguards that are adequate in principle will not be practically sufficient in the face of the terror of an attack, that government officials may use a false emergency as a pretext for oppressive acts, or that social factors like race, religion, or class will influence decision makers.[49] Racial, religious, and class bias have influenced public health responses to epidemics in many instances in our past.[50] We also must be concerned that the breakdown of civil order may include a breakdown of administration in many social institutions, including the court system. The right to challenge a quarantine in court cannot be exercised if there are no court clerks or judges to accept writs or hear cases. In a community cordoned off because of an outbreak of smallpox, there may be no lawyers willing to leave their homes to file cases. Even as states consider the Model Act and make changes to their health codes, it will be important to develop contingency plans and to conduct training within major social institutions such as the judiciary, public health, and medicine. In this sense, the Model Act also attempts to promote the protection of civil liberties by requiring planning and training for a public health emergency.

Drafting and enacting a model emergency health powers act is technically and politically demanding.[51] Law cannot solve all, or even most, of the challenges that would be posed by a catastrophic health event. The nation's public health system is seriously deficient and can be repaired only with sufficient political will and economic resources.[52] Public health agencies must have a robust infrastructure to conduct essential public health services at a level of performance that matches the constantly evolving threats to the health of the public. Critical components of that infrastructure include a well-trained workforce, electronic information and communications systems, rapid disease surveillance and reporting, laboratory, capacity, and emergency response capability.[53] Law is a vital component of the public health infrastructure as well and laws themselves can be highly effective public health interventions. A constitutional democracy must balance the common good with respect for personal dignity, toleration of groups, and adherence to principles of justice.

Funding/Support: The Center for Law and the Public's Health is supported by Cooperative Agreement No. U50/CCU319118–02 from the CDC. The Alfred P. Sloan Foundation provided funding for the development of MSEHPA. The Reforming States Group, composed of leaders of the legislative and executive branches, in collaboration with the Milbank Memorial Fund, provided technical assistance to many states. The MSEHPA grew out of the work of the Public Health Statute Modernization Project of the Robert Wood Johnson Foundation (Turning Point).

Disclaimer: The contents of this article are solely the responsibility of the authors and do not necessarily represent the official views of the CDC or the organizations providing assistance.

Acknowledgment: We gratefully acknowledge the intellectual contributions of many organizations, notably the National Governors Association, National Conference of State Legislatures, National Association of Attorneys General, Association of State and Territorial Health Officials, and National Association of City and County Health Officials. The Public Health Law Program at the CDC offered critical contributions throughout, particularly Richard Goodman, MD, JD, and Gene Matthews, JD. Chai Feldblum, JD, Althea Gregory, JD, Michael Mair, and Julie Muroff, JD, provided research and/or drafting assistance.

NOTES

1. Jernigan JA, Stephens DS, Ashford DA, et al. Bioterrorism-related inhalational anthrax. *Emerg Infect Dis.* 2001;7:933–944.

2. Bush LM, Abrams BH, Beall A, Johnson CC. Index case of fatal inhalations of anthrax due to bioterrorism in the United States. *N Engl J Med.* 2001;345:1607–1610.

3. Inglesby TV, O'Toole T, Henderson DA, et al. Anthrax as a biological weapon, 2002. *JAMA.* 2002;287:2236–2252.

4. Protecting the Homeland: The President's Budget for 2003. Available at: http://www.whitehouse.gov/omb/budget/fy2003/pdf/budO5.pdf. Accessed April 4, 2002.

5. Center for Law and the Public's Health at Georgetown and Johns Hopkins Universities. *The Model State Emergency Health Powers Act.* Washington, DC; 2001. Available at: http://www.publichealthlaw.net. Accessed April 4, 2002.

6. Gostin LO. *Public Health Law: Power, Duty, Restraint.* Berkeley and New York, NY: University of California Press and Milbank Memorial Fund; 2000.

7. Gillis J. States weighing laws to fight bioterrorism. *Washington Post*. November 19, 2001:Al.

8. Lueck S. States seek to strengthen emergency powers: movement is raising privacy and civil-liberties concerns. *Wall Street Journal*. January 7, 2002:A26.

9. Anderson RM, May RM. *Infectious Diseases of Human Dynamics and Control*. New York, NY: Oxford University Press; 1992.

10. Diamond J. *Guns, Germs, and Steel*. New York, NY: WW Norton & Co; 1999.

11. Doebbeling B. Influenza. In: Wallace RB, ed. *Maxcy-Rosenau. Last Public Health and Preventive Medicine*. 14th ed. Stamford, Conn: Appleton & Lange; 1998: 107–112.

12. Anderson RN. *Deaths: Leading Causes for 1999: National Vital Statistics Reports: Volume 49, Number 11*. Hyattsville, Md: National Center for Health Statistics; 2001. Available at: http://www.cdc.gov/nchs/data/nvsr/nvsr49/nvsr49_11.pdf. Accessed April 5, 2002.

13. *The Global Infectious Disease Threat and Its Implications for the United States*. Washington, DC: National Intelligence Council; 2000. Publication NIE 99–17D.

14. US Commission on National Security in the 21st Century. New world coming: American security in the 21st century, supporting research and analysis. September 15, 1999. Available at: http://www.nssg.gov/Reports/reports.htm. Accessed May 31, 2002.

15. Inglesby TV, Henderson DA, Bartlett JG, et al. Anthrax as a biological weapon: medical and public health management. *JAMA*. 1999;281:1735–1745.

16. Inglesby TV, O'Toole T, Henderson DA. Preventing the use of biological weapons: improving response should prevention fail. *Clin Infect Dis*. 2000;30:926–929.

17. Hughes JM. The emerging threat of bioterrorism. *Emerg Infect Dis*. 1999;5: 494–495.

18. Henderson DA. The looming threat of bioterrorism. *Science*. 1999;283: 1279–1282.

19. Cole LA. The specter of biological weapons. *Sci Am*. 1996;275:60–65.

20. Osterholm MT, Schwartz J. *What America Needs to Know to Survive the Coming Bioterrorist Catastrophe*. New York, NY: Bantam Dell; 2001.

21. Cottrell R, Wolffe R. Safe houses yielding documents on weapons of mass destruction. *The Financial Times Limited*. November 23, 2001.

22. O'Toole T, Mair M, Inglesby TV. Shining light on dark winter. *Clin Infect Dis*. 2002;34:972–983.

23. Inglesby TV, Grossman R, O'Toole T. A plague on your city: observations from TOPOFF. *Clin Infect Dis*. 2001;32:436–445.

24. Barbera J, Macintyre A, Gostin L, et al. Large-scale quarantine following biological terrorism in the United States. *JAMA*. 2001;286:2711–2717.

25. Henderson DA. *Testimony Before the Foreign Relations Committee: Hearing on the Threat of Bioterrorism and the Spread of Infectious Disease,* 107th Cong, 1st Sess (September 5, 2001).

26. Gostin LO. *Public Health Law and Ethics: A Reader*. Berkeley and New York, NY: University of California Press and Milbank Memorial Fund; 2002.

27. Gostin LO. Public health law reform. *Am J Public Health.* 2001;91:1365–1368.

28. Colo Rev Stat Ann §24–32–2103 (West 2001).

29. Rhode Island Department of Health. The emergence of bioterrorism as a public health concern in the 21st century: epidemiology and surveillance. Available at: http://www.healthri.org/environment/biot/article.htm. Accessibility verified June 21, 2002.

30. Gostin LO, Burris S, Lazzarini Z. The law and the public's health: a study of infectious disease law in the United States. *Columbia Law Rev.* 1999;99:59–128.

31. Minn Rev Stat Ann §144.419 (West 2002).

32. Institute of Medicine. *Ending Neglect: The Elimination of Tuberculosis in the United States.* Washington, DC: National Academy Press; 2000.

33. Lane HC, Fauci AS. Bioterrorism on the home front: a new challenge for American medicine. *JAMA.* 2001;286:2595–2597.

34, Gostin LO, Lazzarini Z, Neslund VS, Osterholm MT. The public health information infrastructure. *JAMA.* 1996;275:1921–1927.

35. *Public Health Assessment of Potential Biological Terrorism Agents.* Atlanta, Ga: Centers for Disease Control and Prevention; 2002.

36. Horton H, Misrahi JJ, Matthews GW, Kocher PL. Disease reporting as a tool for bioterrorism preparedness. *J Law Med Ethics.* 2002;30:262–266.

37. Kaiser J. Patient privacy: researchers say rules are too restrictive. *Science.* 2001; 294:2070–2071.

38. Cantigny Conference Series. *State Emergency Health Powers and the Bioterrorism Threat.* Chicago, Ill: Cantigny Conference on State Emergency Health Powers and the Bioterrorism Threat; April 26–27, 2001.

39. *Lucas v South Carolina Coastal Council,* 505 US 1003 (1992).

40. Parker-Pope T. Anxious Americans seek antidepressants to cope with terror. *Wall Street Journal.* October 12, 2001:B1.

41. Powell JH. *Bring Out Your Dead: The Great Plague of Yellow Fever in Philadelphia in 1793.* Philadelphia, Pa: University of Pennsylvania Press; 1949.

42. Rosenberg C. *The Cholera Years: The United States 1832, 1839, 1866.* Chicago, Ill: University of Chicago Press; 1987.

43. Novak W. *The People's Welfare: Law and Regulation in Nineteenth Century America.* Chapel Hill and London, NC: University of North Carolina Press; 1996.

44. *Jacobson v Massachusetts,* 197 US 11, 26 (1905).

45. *Commonwealth v Alger,* 7 Cush 53, 84–85 (1851).

46. *Haverly v Bass,* 66 Me 71, 74 (1876).

47. Fidler DP. A globalized theory of public health law. *J Law Med Ethics.* 2002; 30:150–162.

48. Annas G. Bioterrorism, public health, and civil liberties. *N Engl J Med.* 2002; 346:1337–1342.

49. Loff B, Burris S. Compulsory detention: limits of law. *Lancet.* 2001;358:146.

50. Shah N. *Contagious Divides: Epidemics and Race in San Francisco's Chinatown.* Berkeley: University of California Press; 2001.

51. Fox DM. The politics of public health in New York City: contrasting styles since 1920. In: Rosner D, ed. *Hives of Sickness: Public Health and Epidemics in New York City*. New Brunswick, NJ: Rutgers University Press; 1995:197–210.

52. Institute of Medicine. *The Future of Public Health*. Washington, DC: National Academy Press; 1988.

53. *Public Health's Infrastructure: A Status Report: 2001*. Atlanta, Ga: Centers for Disease Control and Prevention; 2002.

5

Collaborating with Industry—Choices for the Academic Medical Center

*Hamilton Moses III, Eugene Braunwald,
Joseph B. Martin, and Samuel O. Thier*

The relationships between academic institutions and private companies are strengthening. The decision of several large pharmaceutical companies, and many biotechnology companies, to build major new laboratories near U.S., European, and Asian universities is just one example of the growing commercial value of academic innovation in biomedicine and the talent that produces it. Individual faculty members and universities in the United States and other countries have increasingly strong financial and nonfinancial incentives to start new companies and to participate directly in the development of drugs, devices, and diagnostic tests.[1]

Many negative implications of this trend have been recognized. Articles in the popular and scientific press have discussed concerns about patient safety in clinical trials, issues related to privacy, conflicts of interest on the part of researchers and their institutions, a shift of priorities in academic research from the public good to private commercial gain, and the potential for disruption of the historical compact between physicians and their patients.[2]

These changes have not gone unnoticed. The Association of American Universities, in collaboration with the Business-Higher Education Forum[3], and the Association of American Medical Colleges (AAMC)[4] have recommended general safeguards and institutional procedures for the management of academic-commercial ties, with special attention to the need to avoid conflicts of interest that may compromise the safety of patients in clinical trials. Several specialty societies have issued recommendations that address particular issues of concern in their fields. Yet these guidelines serve only as starting points for defining what is desirable: they leave many questions unanswered, and they do not address nonclinical research.

THE FORCES CHANGING BIOMEDICAL RESEARCH

Academic biomedical research and industrial biomedical research have similar needs. Both require ready access to specialized talent, from senior investigators through postdoctoral fellows. Researchers from both environments seek interactive, bidirectional relationships that involve the exchange of ideas, materials, and expertise, rather than relationships according to the terms dictated by corporate and university technology-transfer agreements, which emphasize confidentiality, ownership, and valuation of intellectual property. Both groups of scientists often view the university's technology-transfer office and the company's legal staff as barriers to, rather than facilitators of, progress.

The growing scale of research is another important factor that favors collaboration. Basic research in normal biology and disease mechanisms is growing increasingly dependent on sophisticated techniques and complex equipment with high initial costs and high maintenance costs. These expenses are a substantial obstacle for many universities and make industry support or collaboration desirable. On the other hand, the critical task of genotype-phenotype correlation, on which pharmacogenomics, disease-predisposition testing, and early interventions depend, requires access to well-characterized clinical populations and biologic material from normal and affected persons, as well as depth in bioinformatics and computational biology— resources that are the strength of the academic medical center. These complementary forces enhance the interdependence of industry and academic laboratories but also add to difficulties with regard to disclosure, ownership of intellectual property, and the interchange of researchers, information, and biologic materials.

CONFLICTING EXPECTATIONS

Academic medical centers are a public resource. Their different constituencies have competing aspirations, needs, and priorities, creating tensions that are not likely to be eased by simple prescriptive remedies. A number of critical issues are outlined below.

Patients and Their Families

The public expects access to new treatments. Its appetite for innovation has been bolstered by the constant attention given by the press to new treatments and by the implicit promise from researchers of continuing advances. Direct-to-consumer advertising of drugs has increased the public's awareness of new developments in medicine, especially with respect to the treatment of common conditions, with the secondary effect of raising expectations (and health care spending) still further.

Patients demand privacy and control over information about themselves. Information about genetic predisposition is especially troublesome to patient groups and privacy advocates, not only because of the unknown implications for patients and their families, but also because of the fear that once the information proves to be commercially valuable, it will become more difficult to control. These issues led in part to the passage of such legislation as the Health Information Portability and Accountability Act of 1995 and weighed heavily as the act was subsequently modified.[5]

Large and Small Companies (and Their Investors)

The objectives of companies in their relationships to academia often vary according to the size of the company. Large pharmaceutical companies see great value in access to academic talent, ideas, and research tools and deemphasize the importance of discrete inventions and patentable discoveries. In contrast, smaller companies, especially those that develop devices and diagnostic techniques, see greater value in obtaining late-stage technology (i.e., products that are near clinical trial) that are closer to market. These companies derive considerable value from their association with reputable institutions and investigators, which validates their efforts to raise venture capital and the potential value of the company and its product. Venture investors in these entities reinforce the importance of establishing the investigators' full commitment and making it public and visible. The most common vehicle used to assure such commitment is equity or stock options assigned to the investigator and, with increasing frequency, to the institution where the work is performed. Stock or options in young companies are relatively affordable, since they become valuable only if the company and product become successful. Active participation by the investigator in the commercialization process is viewed as essential in creating value. This engenders a powerful but controversial incentive for the investigator and has proved to be one of the most difficult issues for academic centers to manage.

The Press, Legislators, and Regulators

Although many informed persons regard the growing interdependence of universities and commercial entities as necessary if new ideas are to be put into practice, many public advocates are mindful of the need for new rules of engagement that foster the dual goal of innovation and protection of research subjects. All involved parties emphasize, and we agree, that the physician-investigator's and hospital's greatest responsibility is to the welfare of the individual patient and that this responsibility must prevail over all competing interests, including financial gain, reputation building, innovation, economic development, and the demands of entrepreneurs.

CHOICES AND IMPLICATIONS

Given these divergent views and priorities, what are the implications for the academic medical center? We outline seven areas in which critical choices are to be made and discuss how we would face them.

Choice 1: Should Commercial Ties Be Encouraged?

Issues

Academic medical centers vary in the stance they have taken toward commerce. Most universities formally encourage entrepreneurial activity, but informally, local attitudes vary widely. This is not surprising, given the complexity of the tensions between proponents and those who are wary of commercial ties. However, the difference between individual persons' values and the official institutional posture creates uncertainty within the academic community, complicates negotiations with companies, inhibits effective transfer of technology, and is open to misinterpretation by both proponents and skeptics age.

Recommendation

An open, informed, transparent, and timely process must be used to decide the terms of engagement and the protections that are required to prevent conflicts of interest, excessive secrecy (especially so that researchers are free to publish and openly share their findings), and other threats to academic independence. Although the policies of the AAMC, the Association of American Universities, and the National Institutes of Health provide valuable guidelines, they are broad and general and do not effectively address research other than clinical trials. Moreover, the policies leave many questions unanswered, especially the means to implement the guidelines. Therefore, a defined, evenly applied process is required at each academic medical center to answer key questions and to translate policy into practice.

Choice 2: Should Industry Ties Be Managed within the Academic Medical Center?

Issues

Alternative forms of organizations will be required if the full potential of academic-industrial collaboration is to be realized, especially with respect to research in basic biology and disease mechanisms. Such organizations are not new. Several universities have developed free-standing research institutes or foundations to house, manage, and isolate different kinds of research from the main activities of the institution. Examples are the Draper and Lincoln Laboratories and the Whitehead Institute for Biomedical Research, all at the Massachusetts Institute of Technology; the Applied Physics Laboratory at the Johns Hopkins University; and the Wisconsin Alumni Research Foundation of the University of Wisconsin-Madison. Although each of these organizations originally came about for a different reason (to accommodate classified military research, state restrictions, or a donor's preferences), each has proven successful and durable. These free-standing entities have been able to control successfully the two-way flow of personnel and information—into and out of the parent university—without compromising the primary mission of either one.

Several novel public-private collaborations have been formed with the goal of accelerating the pace of basic discovery and its translation into practice. One example is an alliance of the Hereditary Disease Foundation, Aurora Biosciences, and academic researchers of the Huntington Study Group[6] to find new, small-molecule drugs that are effective against Huntington's disease. The foundation provides funding and an organizational structure, and Aurora provides capability in screening of compounds against targets that are identified by the academic researchers. Another example is the Global Alliance for TB Drug Development[7], which was the result of intensive joint effort on the part of the Rockefeller Foundation, the Bill and Melinda Gates Foundation, the World Health Organization, a group of university-based researchers, and several private companies. This alliance seeks to hasten the development of drugs useful against drug-resistant tuberculosis in the developing world. In both of these examples, licensing terms that assured affordability when a drug came to market were explicit at the outset. Both organizations will soon begin clinical trials.

In these alliances, the unique capabilities of the participants are combined to bear on specific problems together, such that obstacles that had stymied previous efforts can be overcome. All of them grew out of the realization that one or two parties could not achieve what they desired without reaching out to others. Each set of relationships overcame critical questions of mutual respect and governance, and their structures allow the control of intellectual property, encouraging free inquiry and supporting the dissemination of new findings, and yet remain compatible with eventual commercialization. Previous attempts at similar alliances have generally failed because they did not agree at the outset on the means to handle these divisive issues.

Recommendation

When specific research goals favor such collaborations, flexible arrangements to accommodate them should be developed. Each approach should be viewed as an experiment and should be subjected to periodic scrutiny and reevaluation of its effectiveness, according to three criteria: whether it furthers academic inquiry, whether it accelerates the development cycle, and whether it has proven manageable.

Choice 3: Should Faculty Be Identified with Companies?

Issues

Among the most troublesome issues is a company's interest in having individual people promote a given product or company openly and visibly, yet maintain a close link to the academic medical center. This practice is potentially dangerous because it blurs the roles of the investigator as an independent agent (a faculty member) and as a partisan (a company representative) and allows the second role to be implicitly linked to the first.

Recommendation

For faculty members who wish to found a company or play an active part in one, increased latitude may best be obtained by taking part-time appointments or leaves of absence. However, a clear separation of academic roles from company roles is essential. Academic medical centers must set a high bar for their faculty, even though such a policy may prove unpopular. In practice, this means that an individual faculty member should be required to choose between making a primary commitment to the company or to the academic medical center; the choice would determine his or her academic title (full-time or adjunct) and roles (e.g., supervision of trainees or ability to accept research funding), without the option to straddle the fence. This approach forces a choice between the relative security afforded by the academic medical center and the hope of rewards in the commercial world. It must be applied to all—from senior, powerful, respected faculty members to junior aspirants.

Choice 4: Should Restrictions on Clinical Research and Basic Research Be Treated Differently?

Issues

The AAMC guidelines provide a helpful framework for policies on clinical trials (effectively proscribing any financial interest on the part of an investigator of a drug), but they leave ambiguity about devices and are silent on basic, nonclinical research. They also do not clarify the gray zone of translational, disease-focused research that relies on human tissue and clinical information but does not involve testing of patients or volunteers.

Recommendation

We propose the adoption of very specific working definitions of clinical research and basic research. Whether research is or is not clinical can be determined according to the need for approval from an institutional review board for its conduct. This establishes a clear definition, one that would include essentially all investigations requiring human tissue, clinical information and records, or contact with patients, and not just clinical trials. For basic research not requiring institutional review board approval, academic medical centers may offer greater latitude to the researcher who wishes to conduct commercial research in which he or she has a financial interest. However, since federal policy has inexorably expanded the purview of institutional review boards, progressively less research involving patients, patient information, and tissue will be exempt.

Choice 5: Should Devices Be Treated as a Special Case?

Issues

The development and evaluation of medical devices have proven to be a contentious issue in past discussions, and ones in which both dangers and potential benefits are palpable. The AAMC guidelines leave substantial uncertainty about how the case-by-case decisions they support should be applied.

Recommendation

We propose that the same standard be adopted for both drugs and devices, by precluding physician-inventors from evaluating their device or procedure. In special cases, it may be desirable to have the initial clinical use of a device performed by the physician-inventor, but only under careful and prospectively defined oversight by persons who are at arm's length. Only independent investigators who have no ties to the inventor should select patients and assess safety, efficacy, and long-term outcomes; for this reason, the investigators and the inventors will need to be based at different institutions. We advocate making a clear distinction between device development and device evaluation. Physician-inventors should usually be involved in the early stages of prototype refinement and of the first use of a device in patients but must not have influence over its subsequent evaluation. This policy will ensure independence and reduce real and perceived conflicts. It will also increase the generalizability and broad acceptance of the technique or device, if it is shown to be effective.

Choice 6: How Is the Proper Balance between Commercially Sponsored Research and Government or Foundation Research to Be Achieved?

Issues

It is striking that many of the fears expressed today about undue dependence on industry were invoked in the 1950s about the nascent National Institutes of Health and the growing reliance of research on government.[8] Fifty years later, it is clear that U.S. academic medical centers owe their current scientific productivity, diversity, organization, and size to the decade-by-decade expansion of federally funded research.

Recommendation

All research should be judged by the same yardstick: whether it will further the aims of discovery, innovation, and productivity and not solely serve financial aspirations. Academic investigators may need to be very selective and to seek preferentially partners in industry who understand and desire two-way interactions and are willing to be flexible in managing the terms of engagement, the inevitable conflicts over intellectual-property claims, and the other issues that arise. Investigators will need to seek partners who understand and respect the priorities of academic research and who can live with them.

Choice 7: How Should Institutional Conflicts of Interest Be Managed?

Issues

When an academic medical center itself has financial interest in a company, questions about its independence of judgment and oversight may arise, especially with respect to clinical research. Implicit is the question, "Can the fox guard the chickens?" This is among the most vexing of questions, one in regard to which the AAMC has offered especially helpful guidance.

Recommendation

The AAMC framework for deciding whether a conflict exists should be adopted, and when a conflict arises, all of its financial aspects should be managed by a separate entity at arm's length, with oversight by persons not affiliated with the academic medical center. Implied in this approach is the isolation of the institutional review board from any responsibility for managing conflicts of interest. Although the institutional review board must be made aware of conflicts of interest and of any relationships that an investigator has that may give rise to such conflicts, the board should have responsibility solely for patient protection. To identify unacceptable conflicts, proscribe clinical research that is subject to conflicts, and ensure that another independent entity is overseeing institutional conflicts are sufficient responsibilities for an institutional review board.

CONCLUSIONS

A decade ago, our own institutions adopted conservative positions on the questions we pose here. Among the most controversial of these has been the proscription of personal financial ties between sponsoring companies and basic-science investigators who receive research funding from them. More proscriptively, Harvard Medical School does not allow a clinical investigator to accept research support from a company in which he or she holds equity, has an executive position, serves as a director or key advisor, or receives more than minimal consulting fees.

Other institutions face the same choices; many will take different positions. Given the potential value of collaboration, the current national attention to ethics in business, and the considerable risk to the trust patients place in their doctors, we must continually re-evaluate our approaches. Although policies will vary, we think some policies—separation of institutional review boards

from economic influences, management of institutional and personal conflicts at arm's length, and consistent treatment of all faculty members, regardless of rank—must be immutable. In the words of one senior observer,
"We must get this right, or we will all lose in the process."

HAMILTON MOSES III, M.D. Boston Consulting Group, Bethesda, MD 20814

EUGENE BRAUNWALD, M.D. Partners HealthCare System, Boston, MA 02199

JOSEPH B. MARTIN, M.D., PH.D. Harvard Medical School, Boston, MA 02115

SAMUEL O. THIER, M.D. Partners HealthCare System, Boston, MA 02199

Dr. Moses, a senior advisor at the Boston Consulting Group, has reported that
he actively consults with academic medical centers and pharmaceutical and
biotechnology companies in the United States, Europe, and Asia. Dr. Braunwald has reported that his group receives research support from Bristol-
Myers Squibb, Aventis, Merck, Millennium, and British Biotech. Dr. Martin
has reported that he is a member of the boards of directors of Baxter Healthcare, Cytyc, and Scientific Learning. Dr. Thier has reported that he is on the
boards of directors of Merck, Charles River Laboratories, and Pranalytica (a
medical-device company).

Drs. Braunwald, Martin, and Thier, listed alphabetically, contributed
equally to this article.

We are indebted to Heidi Model, Massachusetts General Hospital, Boston.

NOTES

1. Kennedy D. Enclosing the research commons. Science 2001;294:2249.

2. Kelch RP. Maintaining the public trust in clinical research. N Engl J Med
2002;346:285–7

3. The Business-Higher Education Forum. Working together, creating knowledge:
University-Industry Research Collaboration Initiative. Washington, D.C.: American
Council on Education, 2001.

4. Task Force on Financial Conflicts of Interest in Clinical Research. Protecting
subjects, preserving trust and promoting progress: policy and guidelines for the oversight of individual financial interests in research. Washington, D.C.: Association of
American Medical Colleges, December 2001. (Accessed October 4, 2002, at
http://www.aamc.org/ members/coitf/start.htm.)

5. Kulynych J, Korn D. The effect of the new federal medical-privacy rule on research. N Engl J Med 2002;346:201–4.

6. The HDF partners with Aurora Biosciences for therapeutic drug discovery. Santa Monica, Calif.: Hereditary Disease Foundation, September 2000. (Accessed October 4, 2002, at http://www.hdfoundation.org/news.html.)

7. Development of new anti-TB treatments affordable in worst hit countries is aim of new, global public-private partnership. New York: Global Alliance for TB Drug Development, October 10, 2000. (Accessed October 4, 2002, at http://www. stoptb.org/Working_Groups/alliance/pressrelease. html.)

8. Starr P. The social transformation of American medicine. New York: Basic Books, 1982:338–44.

6

The Continuing Unethical Conduct of Underpowered Clinical Trials

Scott D. Halpern, Jason H. T. Karlawish, and Jesse A. Berlin

Despite long-standing critiques of the conduct of underpowered clinical trials, the practice not only remains widespread, but also has garnered increasing support. Patients and healthy volunteers continue to participate in research that may be of limited clinical value, and authors recently have offered 2 related arguments to support the validity and value of underpowered clinical trials: that meta-analysis may "save" small studies by providing a means to combine the results with those of other similar studies to enable estimates of an intervention's efficacy, and that although small studies may not provide a good basis for testing hypotheses, they may provide valuable estimates of treatment effects using confidence intervals. In this article, we examine these arguments in light of the distinctive moral issues associated with the conduct of underpowered trials, the disclosures that are owed to potential participants in underpowered trials so they may make autonomous enrollment decisions, and the circumstances in which the prospects for future meta-analyses may justify individually underpowered trials. We conclude that underpowered trials are ethical in only 2 situations: small trials of interventions for rare diseases in which investigators document explicit plans for including their results with those of similar trials in a prospective meta-analysis, and early-phase trials in the development of drugs or devices, provided they are adequately powered for defined purposes other than randomized treatment comparisons. In both cases, investigators must inform prospective subjects that their participation may only indirectly contribute to future health care benefits.

More than 20 years have passed since investigators first described the ethical problems of conducting randomized controlled trials (RCTS) with insufficient statistical power.[1, 2] Because such studies may not adequately test the underlying hypotheses, they have been considered "scientifically useless"[2] and therefore unethical in their exposure of participants to the risks and burdens of human research.[2-4] Despite this long-standing challenge, many clinical investigators continue to conduct underpowered studies[5, 6] and fail to calculate or report appropriate (a priori) power analyses.[6-10] Not only do these scientific and ethical errors persist in the general medical literature, but 3 recent reports[11-13] also highlight the alarming prevalence of these problems in more specialized fields.

Patients and healthy volunteers thus continue to participate in research that may be of limited clinical value.[4, 14] Furthermore, authors[15-17] recently have offered 2 related arguments to support the validity and value of underpowered clinical trials. First, meta-analysis may "save" small studies by providing a means to combine the results with those of other similar studies to enable estimates of an interventions efficacy. Second, although small studies may not provide a good basis for testing hypotheses, they may provide valuable estimates of treatment effects using confidence intervals. Based on these arguments, authors have suggested that institutional review boards (IRBS) drop the documentation of statistical power as a criterion for study approval.[16]

If meta-analysis and estimating treatment effects provided investigators and IRBs with a means to justify underpowered research, challenges to the ethics of underpowered studies would have to cease. In this article, we examine these arguments in light of the distinctive moral issues associated with the conduct of underpowered trials, the disclosures that are owed to potential participants in underpowered trials so they may make autonomous enrollment decisions, and the circumstances in which the prospects for future meta-analyses may justify individually underpowered trials.

We conclude that underpowered trials can be ethical in only 2 situations. First, small trials of interventions for rare diseases may be justified if investigators document explicit plans for including their results with those of similar trials in a prospective meta-analysis. Second, early-phase trials in the development of drugs, devices, or other interventions need not be powered to make randomized treatment comparisons provided they are adequately powered for other defined purposes and designed to guide the conduct of subsequent, comparative trials. In both cases, investigators must inform prospective participants that their participation may only indirectly contribute to future health care benefits.

STATISTICAL POWER AND THE PLANNING OF CLINICAL TRIALS

Investigators use power analysis to determine the probability that a given study will reject the null hypothesis when it is, in fact, false. In other words, power analysis determines the chance of detecting a true-positive result. By tradition, researchers consider a study to be adequately powered if it has at least an 80% chance of detecting a clinically significant effect when one exists. This exact value is arbitrary; higher power will always be preferable and should be set with consideration of the importance of limiting both false-negative conclusions (ie, type II errors) and false-positive conclusions (ie, type I errors).

To calculate a study's power to detect a given effect, investigators use a set of other variables, including the number of individuals to be enrolled, the expected variability of their outcomes, and the chosen probability of making a type I error. Reformulating these variables allows one to calculate the numbers of study participants needed to detect a clinically important effect size with acceptable power. Although consensus among reasonable clinicians will generally enable determinations of how small an effect would be clinically important to detect, disagreement about this value may occasionally emerge. In such cases, we advocate a 3-tiered, hierarchical approach for investigators to use in determining the effect size to be entered into sample size calculations.

First, when empirical definitions of clinically meaningful effects exist, such as in the percentage reduction of reported pain necessary to define analgesic efficacy,[18] these values ought to be used. Second, if there is neither clinical consensus nor empirical evidence to guide definitions of clinically important effects, but data from earlier trials or observational studies reliably indicate an intervention's plausible effect, this value may be used. Finally, if none of the foregoing criteria are met, then previously published definitions of moderate effect sizes, such as those described by Cohen[19], should be used. Trials that cannot reliably detect effect sizes defined using this hierarchical approach may be defined as underpowered.

ARGUMENTS FOR ALLOWING UNDERPOWERED TRIALS

There are several practical barriers to conducting large RCTS, particularly for rare diseases. Because the results of smaller, underpowered trials may later be combined in meta-analyses, authors have argued that prohibiting underpowered trials would "thwart many independent investigations . . . [which] may seriously diminish the stock of the world's knowledge."[16] There are both practical and ethical problems with this argument.

The first practical problem stems from an overly optimistic view of the usefulness of the information that underpowered trials may provide. Acknowledging that hypothesis tests are inordinately likely to produce false-negative results when inadequately powered, proponents argue that quantifying the range of plausible effect sizes will still be possible by examining confidence intervals.[16] However, studies containing too few subjects to detect a positive effect (if one exists) via hypothesis testing will also yield unacceptably wide confidence intervals around the point estimate of this effect. Because such confidence intervals will often contain both the null and clinically important effect sizes, the approach provides ambiguous conclusions.

One might argue that if no trials were conducted, the confidence intervals around the (unknown) effect would remain infinitely wide. Thus, any well-designed trial, no matter how small, would at least reduce this uncertainty. However, the marginal value of narrowing confidence intervals to widths still compatible with both positive and negative results generally is insufficient to justify exposing individuals to the common risks and burdens of research. Although these risks and burdens may often be outweighed by the benefits of trial participation,[20] these beneficial effects are not uniform,[20] and their potential is insufficient to justify human research.[14]

The second practical problem with meta-analysis is that even if investigators conducted multiple underpowered trials, difficulties in synthesizing the results may prevent the calculation of valid treatment effects. Under ideal conditions, meta-analyses offer potential advantages over a single RCT in gauging a treatment effect. Meta-analyses may enhance generalizability by incorporating more heterogeneous populations and may overcome the risk that any single RCT, even a very large one, could be weakened by bias.

For meta-analyses to be useful, however, comparable research methods must have been used among the primary trials, and these trials must be selected for inclusion in an unbiased fashion. The infrequency with which these ideal conditions are met may help explain why 2 independent meta-analyses of the same literature sometimes arrive at different conclusions.[21, 22] As Bailar notes, "Such disagreement argues powerfully against any notion that meta-analysis offers an assured way to distill the 'truth' from a collection of research papers."[22]

Finally, because underpowered trials are more likely to produce negative results and consequently may not be published (the so-called publication bias[23, 24]), underpowered trials may be less accessible for inclusion in meta-analyses.[25] This may fatally bias the approach. Thus, the ideal conditions for combining evidence may be particularly unlikely when the component trials are underpowered; therefore, even the most rigorously conducted meta-analyses will be unable to augment such trials' abilities to further medical knowledge. Only if widely accessible registries of RCTs[26, 27] are expanded to include privately sponsored trials could the potential for publication bias in retrospective meta-analyses be eliminated.[28]

SAMPLE SIZE AND INFORMED CONSENT

In addition to the practical problems mentioned herein, underpowered studies will also be ethically deficient if investigators do not convey these studies' limited value to prospective participants. Failure to communicate a study's value (or lack thereof) limits the quality of the information on which individuals must base their enrollment decisions. Individuals commonly participate in research to fulfill altruistic motives, such as desires to advance medical science and thereby help others.[29–35] Therefore, to respect prospective participants' autonomy, investigators must inform them of the limited capacities of small trials to produce public benefit.

Investigators occasionally deprive participants of such information for 3 reasons. First, investigators may simply fail to conduct an a priori power analysis. Such investigators are acting negligently. In addition to risking the enrollment of too few participants to answer the research question, investigators who fail to conduct or improperly conduct a power analysis may enroll too many individuals. This outcome is also troubling because it exposes too many individuals to the risks of research and overconsumes limited societal resources.[2, 36, 37]

Second, investigators might conduct an appropriate power calculation but fail to recruit sufficient numbers of participants in a timely fashioner.[38, 39] Such cases may arise, for example, when prospective participants' clinicians have reservations about enrolling their patients[40] or when patients themselves are dissuaded by some feature of the trial, such as the existence of a placebo group.[34, 41] Investigators should attempt to identify potential recruitment problems beforehand and modify their approaches accordingly.[42]

Perhaps most concerning is the third scenario, in which investigators conduct an appropriate power analysis, find they will be unlikely to recruit an adequate number of participants, and choose to proceed without conveying this information to participants in the informed consent process. This knowing failure of information disclosure entails deception. In addition to abrogating participants' rights, if such deception were publicized, it could undermine people's trust in science, further curtailing future enrollment.

Investigators may fear that disclosing information regarding power will itself reduce enrollment. Because study participants so often seek to fulfill altruistic Motives[29–35, 43] it seems logical that they would rather participate in adequately powered trials. Nonetheless, this potential barrier to efficient recruitment does not justify enrolling individuals without full disclosure.

RARE DISEASES

For research on diseases with low prevalence or incidence, the numbers of afflicted (or newly afflicted) individuals at any one time may make it impossible to conduct even a multi-center RCT that could reliably distinguish between interventions. It has been argued that in such cases some evidence is better than none.[16, 17] This view ignores the fact that only when the effect sizes are extremely large—indeed, larger than anticipated—will small trials be able serendipitously to document them. In all other cases, false-negative conclusions may be drawn and post hoc power analyses will be unable to elucidate the error.[44] Although investigators commonly relax inferential standards to avoid this result, doing so increases the risk of drawing false-positive conclusions.

Instead, if investigators explicitly plan to make the results of a small trial available for inclusion in a prospective meta-analysis, excessive risks of both types of false conclusions may be averted. Prospectively designed meta-analyses are less susceptible to the problems with traditional, retrospective meta-analyses because the methods of the component studies may be synchronized in advance. This avoids the possibility that component studies may not be combinable if, for example, one study investigated a high-dose intervention among men and another study investigated a lower dose of the intervention among women.[45] Because dose and sex would be inextricably confounded between these studies, retrospective meta-analysis would be of little use.

Therefore, only prospectively designed meta-analyses can justify the risks to participants in individually underpowered trials because they provide sufficient assurance that a study's results will eventually contribute to valuable or important knowledge.[46] Although a multicenter trial could similarly contribute to generalizable knowledge and may provide more internally valid results, it requires that investigators have access to a sufficient number of patients during the trial's conduct. This may not be possible for very rare diseases, making prospective meta-analyses of single-center and multicenter trials necessary to obtain adequate power. Furthermore, prospectively designed meta-analyses retain the innovation possible in conducting several smaller studies, while providing the organizational framework to ensure that their results can be synthesized.

EARLY-PHASE STUDIES OF EXPERIMENTAL INTERVENTIONS

Just as prospective meta-analyses may ensure the value of small single studies for rare diseases, plans for large, comparative trials of experimental interventions can justify the conduct of small studies in earlier phases of drug or device development. Thus, several smaller phase 1/2 trials may be justified as long as each is adequately powered for another aim, such as reliably determining whether a new therapy shows at least some promise of benefit, and is explicitly aimed at guiding a definitive phase 3 trial that will be adequately powered to make a reliable treatment comparison. Investigators conducting these studies must tell participants that their participation will not directly provide information of immediate clinical value, but rather will guide future studies that may do so.

CONCLUSION

Despite long-standing critiques of the conduct of underpowered clinical trials, the practice not only remains widespread, but also has garnered increasing support. We have provided 2 main arguments for why these trends cannot be ethically reconciled. First, failing to conduct a priori power analyses fails to respect participants' decision-making autonomy by limiting the information disclosed during the informed consent process. Second, proceeding with underpowered trials, in the absence of explicit plans for definitive studies in the future, shifts the risk-benefit calculus that helps justify research in an unfavorable direction.[14] Participants in such trials experience personal risks and benefits commensurate with those in adequately powered trials, but are denied the same opportunity to contribute to the improved care of future patients. Therefore, IRB members should carefully monitor the statements made in the consent forms regarding the potential benefits of participation to ensure that these statements accurately reflect the strength of the underlying study design.

Low statistical power is merely one manifestation of a much larger problem: that many clinical investigators are not properly trained in research methods. The consequences are not only that investigators fail to properly assess the required sample size. Poor training may also explain why investigators may improperly assess the state of knowledge before initiating new studies, fail to appreciate how new trials ought to be conducted to advance this knowledge, choose inappropriate end points, and poorly report the results of their work.

We have focused our discussion on power because it remains one prominent problem, both scientifically and ethically, for which a workable solution is possible. We recommend that investigators always conduct a priori power calculations and relay the results to potential study participants. This should not be an overwhelming task. Simplified statements regarding both the inherent uncertainty in all research and whether the relative level of uncertainty in the proposed study conforms to standards of clinical investigation should be understandable by potential participants.

After conveying information in this way, the research must still meet one of the following conditions: either enough patients will be enrolled to obtain at least 80% power to detect a clinically important effect or, if this is not possible, the researchers will be able to document a clear and practical plan to integrate the results of their trial with those of future trials. Absent one of these 2 circumstances, ethics review boards, research funding agencies, and medical journal editors should maintain strict requirements for adequate research methods, including appropriate statistical power, for any clinical trial to be approved, funded, or published, respectively.

Author Contributions: *Study concept and design*: Halpern, Karlawish, Berlin.
Drafting of the manuscript: Halpern.
Critical revision of the manuscript for important intellectual content: Halpern, Karlawish, Berlin.
Statistical expertise: Berlin.
Study supervision: Karlawish, Berlin.
Funding/Support: Mr Halpern is supported by a pre-doctoral fellowship from the American Heart Association, Dallas, Tex, and a National Research Service Award in Cardiopulmonary Epidemiology from the National Heart, Lung, and Blood Institute, Bethesda, Md. Dr Kadawish is supported by a Brookdale National Fellowship, a National Institute on Aging Mentored Clinical Scientist Development Award, and a Paul Beeson Fellowship.
Acknowledgment: We thank Jon F. Merz, JD, PhD, and Kathleen Joy Propert, ScD, for their insightful comments on an early version of the manuscript.

NOTES

1. Newell DJ. Type II errors and ethics. *BMJ*. 1978;4:1789.

2. Altman DG. Statistics and ethics in medical research III: how large a sample? *BMJ*. 1980;281:1336–1338.

3. Rutstein DD. The ethical design of human experiments. In: Freund PA, ed. *Experimentation With Human Subjects*. New York, NY: George Braziller; 1970: 383–401.

4. Freedman B. Scientific value and validity as ethical requirements for research: a proposed explication. *IRB Rev Hum Subjects Res*. 1987;9:7–10.

5. Freiman JA, Chalmers TC, Smith H Jr, Kuebler RR. The importance of beta, the type II error and sample size in the design and interpretation of the randomized controlled trial: survey of 71 "negative" trials. *N Engl J Med*. 1978;299:690–694.

6. Moher D, Dulberg CS, Wells GA. Statistical power, sample size, and their reporting in randomized controlled trials. *JAMA*. 1994;272:122–124.

7. DerSimonian R, Charette LJ, McPeek B, Mosteller F. Reporting on methods in clinical trials. *N Engl J Med*. 1982;306:1332–1337.

8. Pocock SJ, Hughes MD, Lee RJ. Statistical problems in the reporting of clinical trials. *N Engl J Med*. 1987;317:426–432.

9. Altman DG, Dore CJ. Randomization and base-line comparisons in clinical trials. *Lancet* 1990;335:149–153.

10. Schumm LP, Fisher JS, Thisted RA, Olak J. Clinical trials in general surgical journals: are methods better reported? *Surgery*. 1999;125:41–45.

11. Nichol MB, Venturini F, Sung JC. A critical evaluation of the methodology of the literature on medication compliance. *Ann Pharmacother*. 1999;33:531–535.

12. Freedman KB, Bernstein J. Sample size and statistical power in clinical orthopaedic research. *J Bone Joint Surg Am*. 1999;81:1454–1460.

13. Dickinson K, Bunn F, Wentz R, Edwards P, Roberts I. Size and quality of randomised controlled trials in head injury: review of published studies. *BMJ*. 2000; 320:1308–1311.

14. Emmanuel EJ, Wendler D, Grady C. What makes clinical research ethical? *JAMA*. 2000;283:2701–2711.

15. Chalmers TC, Lau J. Meta-analytic stimulus for changes in clinical trials. *Stat Methods Med Res*. 1993; 2:161–172.

16. Edwards SJL, Lilford RJ, Braunholtz D, Jackson J. Why "underpowered" trials are not necessarily unethical. *Lancet*. 1997;350:804–807.

17. Knapp TR. The overemphasis on power analysis. *Nursing Res*. 1996;45: 379–381.

18. Farrar JT, Portenoy RK, Berlin JA, Kinman J, Strom BL. Defining the clinically important difference in pain outcome measures. *Pain*. 2000;88:287–294.

19. Cohen J. *Statistical Power Analysis for the Behavioral Sciences*. 2nd ed. Hillsdale, NJ: Lawrence Erlbaum; 1988.

20. Braunholtz DA, Edwards SJL, Lilford RJ. Are randomized clinical trials good for us (in the short term)? evidence for a "trial effect." *Clin Epidemiol*. 2001; 54:217–224.

21. Simes JR. Prospective meta-analysis of cholesterol-lowering studies: the Prospective Pravastatin Pooling (PPP) Project and the Cholesterol Treatment Trialists (CTT) Collaboration. *Am J Cardiol* 1995;76:122C–126C.

22. Bailar JC. The promise and problems of meta-analysis. *N Engl J Med*. 1997;337:559–561.

23. Begg CB, Berlin JA. Publication bias: a problem in interpreting medical data. *J R Stat Soc A*. 1988; 151:419–463.

24. Egger M, Smith GD. Meta-analysis: bias in location and selection of studies. *BMJ*. 1998;316:61–66.

25. Matthews JNS. Small clinical trials: are they all bad? *StatMed*. 1995;14:115–126.

26. Current Controlled Trials Ltd. Current Controlled Trials. Available at: http://www.controlledtrials.com. Accessibility verified October 29, 2001.

84 Halpern, Karlawish, and Berlin

27. National Institutes of Health. ClinicalTrials.gov. Available at: http://clinicaltrials. gov. Accessibility verified October 29, 2001.

28. Horton R, Smith R. Time to register randomised trials. *BMJ.* 1999; 319:865–866.

29. Cassileth BR, Lusk EJ, Miller DS, Hurwitz S. Attitudes toward clinical trials among patients and the public. *JAMA.* 1982;248:968–970.

30. Mattson ME, Curb JD, McArdle R, and the AMIS and BHAT Research Groups. Participation in a clinical trial: the patients' point of view. *Control Clin Trials.* 1985;6:156–167.

31. Schron EB, Wassertheil-Smoller S, Pressel S, for the SHEP Cooperative Research Group. Clinical trial participant satisfaction: survey of SHEP enrollees. *J Am Geriatr Soc.* 1997;45:934–938.

32. Koblin BA, Heagerty P, Sheon A, et al. *Readiness of high-risk populations in the HIV Network for Prevention Trials to participate in HIV vaccine efficacy trials in the United States.* AIDS. 1998;12:785–793.

33. Sugarman J, Kass NE, Goodman SN, Perentesis P, Fernandes P, Faden RR. What patients say about medical research. *IRB Rev Hum Subjects Res.* 1998; 20:1–7.

34. Welton AJ, Vickers MR, Cooper JA, Meade TW, Marteau TM. Is recruitment more difficult with a placebo arm in randomised controlled trials? a quasirandomised, interview based study. *BMJ.* 1999;318:1114–1117.

35. Karlawish JHT, Casarett D, Klocinski J, Sankar P. How do Alzheimer's disease patients and their caregivers decide whether to enroll in a clinical trial? *Neurology.* 2001;56:789–792,

36. Altman DG. The scandal of poor medical research. *BMJ.* 1994;308:283–284.

37. Knottnerus JA, Bouter LM. The ethics of sample size: two-sided testing and one-sided thinking. J *Clin Epidemiol.* 2001;54:109–110.

38. Hunninghake DB, Darby CA, Probstfield JL. Recruitment experience in clinical trials: literature summary and annotated bibliography. *Control Clin Trials.* 1987;8 (suppl 4):6S-30S.

39. Meinert CL. Patient recruitment and enrollment. In: *Clinical Trials: Design, Conduct and Analysis.* New York, NY: Oxford University Press; 1986:149–158.

40. Taylor KM, Margolese RG, Soskolne CL. Physicians' reasons for not entering eligible patients in a randomized clinical trial of adjuvant surgery for breast cancer. *N Engl J Med.* 1984;310:1363–1367.

41. Feagan BG, Fedorak RN, Irvine EJ, et al. A comparison of methotrexate with placebo for the maintenance of remission in Crohn's disease. *N Engl J Med.* 2000;342:1627–1632.

42. Halpern SD, Metzger DS, Berlin JA., Ubel PA. Who will enroll? predicting participation in a phase 11 AIDS vaccine trial. *J Acquir Immune Defic Syndr.* 2001;27: 281–288.

43. Freedman B. Suspended judgement: AIDS and the ethics of clinical trials: learning the right lessons. *Control Clin Trials.* 1992;13:1–5.

44. Goodman SN, Berlin JA. The use of predicted confidence intervals when planning experiments and the misuse of power when interpreting results. *Ann Intern Med.* 1994;121;200–206.

45. Berlin JA, Colditz GA. The role of meta-analysis in the regulatory process for foods, drugs, and devices. *JAMA*. 1999;281:830–834.

46. Department of Health and Human Services. Common rule (45 CFR §46). Federal policy for the protection of human subjects; notices and rules. 1991:28003–28032.

7

Effect of Mandatory Parental Notification on Adolescent Girls' Use of Sexual Health Care Services

Diane M. Reddy, Raymond Fleming, and Carolyne Swain

Context Mandatory parental notification for adolescents to obtain prescribed contraceptives is a controversial issue. Recently, legislation that would prohibit prescribed contraceptives for adolescents without parental involvement was introduced in 10 states and the US Congress.

Objective To determine the effect of mandatory parental notification for prescribed contraceptives on use of sexual health care services by adolescent girls.

Design, Setting, and Participants Girls younger than 18 years and seeking services at all 33 Planned Parenthood family planning clinics in Wisconsin (n=1118) were surveyed during the spring of 1999. A response rate of 85% was achieved, yielding a sample of 950 girls.

Main Outcome Measures Percentages of girls who reported that they would stop using all sexual health care services, delay testing or treatment for human immunodeficiency virus (HIV) or other sexually transmitted diseases (STDs) or discontinue using specific (but not all) services because of parental notification.

Results Fifty-nine percent (n=556) indicated they would stop using all sexual health care services, delay testing or treatment for HIV or other STDs, or discontinue use of specific (but not all) sexual health care services if their parents were informed that they were seeking prescribed contraceptives. Eleven percent indicated that they would discontinue or delay STD texts or treatment, even though the survey made it clear that mandatory parental notification would occur only for prescribed contraceptives. Analysis comparing girls of different ages and races and from urban vs rural clinics showed that, although the 17–year-olds and African American girls were significantly less

likely to stop using sexual health care services with mandatory parental notification, roughly half of the 17–year-olds (56%) and African American girls
(49%) indicated that they would stop using all sexual health care services, delay testing or treatment for HIV or other STDs, or discontinue use of specific
(but not all) services with mandatory parental notification.

Conclusion Mandatory parental notification for prescribed contraceptives
would impede girls' use of sexual health care services, potentially increasing
teen pregnancies and the spread of STDs.

Mandatory parental notification for adolescents obtaining prescribed contraceptives is a controversial issue. Proponents argue that requiring parental notification would strengthen parents' ability to educate their children and safeguard them from the medical risks associated with prescribed contraceptives.
Some proponents also believe that mandating parental notification would encourage adolescents to use condoms rather than prescribed contraceptives, reducing rates of sexually transmitted diseases (STDs).

In 1998, Congress considered the Title X Parental Notification Act requiring written parental consent, a court order, or parental notification 5 business
days in advance of providing minors with prescribed contraceptives at all US
family planning clinics funded under Title X of the Public Health Services
Act. More recently, efforts have been made to bar the use of state matching
funds to purchase prescription drugs for minors without parental consent and
to deny federal public health and education funds to all school districts offer-
ing emergency contraception in school-based health centers without parental
consent. In addition, within the last 5 years, at least 10 states have introduced
bills to mandate parental involvement in girls' access to prescribed contraceptives. When state law permits or requires parental notification, the new
federal medical privacy regulations issued in December 2000 regarding use
and disclosure of health information defers to state law.[1] Given these parental
involvement proposals and recent legislation concerning other reproductive
health care issues, other proposals prohibiting prescribed contraceptives for
sexually active adolescent girls without parental notification are likely.

Although professional medical organizations strongly encourage and support parental involvement in adolescents' sexual health care decisions, they
also recognize the importance of confidential contraceptive services and STD
testing and treatment in curbing the high incidence and prevalence of pregnancies and STDs. As far back as 1967, the American Medical Association
(AMA) took the position that minors should be able to be tested and treated
for STDs without parental notification.[2] In the 1970s, 1980s, and 1990s, the
AMA opposed legislation requiring parental involvement for adolescents to

obtain prescribed contraceptives, and in 1988 the American College of Obstetricians and Gynecologists, the American Academy of Pediatrics, the American Academy of Family Physicians, and the National Medical Association concluded that "ultimately, the health risks to adolescents are so impelling that legal barriers in deference to parental involvement should not stand in the way of needed care."[3] Furthermore, the AMA National Coalition on Adolescent Health reaffirmed the need for confidential sexual health care services for adolescents[4], and the AMA Council on Scientific Affairs urged members to actively oppose legislation requiring parental consent or notification that would impede health care.[5] In sum, professional medical organizations have taken a firm stand against mandatory parental involvement regulations for prescribed contraceptives and STD tests and treatment.

Although research[6] examining the general issue of adolescent attitudes about parental involvement in their seeking of health care found that less than 20% of adolescents were willing to seek health care for birth control, pregnancy, or an STD with parental involvement, the only studies to directly assess whether mandatory parental notification would change the behavior of adolescent girls using contraceptive services were conducted more than 20 years ago.[7, 8] One study was a regional survey (n = 1442), and the other was a national survey (n = 1211). Thirty-six percent of adolescent girls in the regional survey and 23% of those in the national survey reported that if parental notification were required, they would stop using sexual health care services. These figures may be underestimates. In both surveys, girls were asked whether their parents knew they were seeking prescribed contraceptives before they were asked whether parental notification would cause them to stop using services. Asking the question, "Do your parents know?" may have prompted some girls to say yes out of a desire to make sure they would get prescribed contraceptives, even though their parents might not know. In addition, in the national survey, 5% of girls said they were unsure whether their parents knew they were seeking prescribed contraceptives. What these girls would do if parental notification were required is unaccounted for. Further, in both surveys, whether parental notification would cause girls to stop using family planning services was the only outcome assessed. Other plausible outcomes, such as discontinuing use of specific (but not all) sexual health services or delaying testing or treatment for human immunodeficiency virus (HIV) or other STDs, were not investigated. Therefore, the impact of mandatory parental notification may have been even greater than the estimates provided by these 2 surveys.

Sexually active adolescent girls using family planning services may have become more or less concerned about mandatory parental notification for obtaining prescribed contraceptives throughout the past 2 decades. Consequently, this statewide survey was conducted to investigate whether mandatory parental notification for prescribed contraceptives would cause girls to stop using sexual health care services, delay testing or treatment for HIV or other STDs, or discontinue their use of specific (but not all) sexual health services.

METHODS

Participants in the Statewide Sample

The data were collected from all Planned Parenthood family planning clinics in Wisconsin (n = 33) in the spring of 1999. All single, sexually active girls who were younger than 18 years and presented to the clinics (n = 1118) were asked to complete a confidential institutional review board-approved survey. Fifteen percent declined, primarily because of time constraints. A total of 950 sexually active adolescent girls voluntarily completed the survey. The participants were a mean 16.8 years of age (SD, 1.06; range, 12–17 years). The sample was 79.9% white, 13.5% African American, 2.6% Hispanic, 2.4% Asian, and 0.9% Native American. The remaining (0.7%) indicated multiple ethnic heritage.

Several steps were taken to ensure that the survey questions were valid. Established principles of survey development were used to construct the survey. The survey was extensively evaluated and pilot tested to ensure that the questions were clear, the wording was at a fifth-grade reading level, and the format facilitated completion. To enhance the validity of responses, girls were assured that the survey would not include specific information that could identify them.

Adolescents were asked by clinic staff to complete the confidential survey individually as they waited for their appointments. Clinic staff instructed girls to answer each item honestly and answered any questions the adolescents posed. The completed surveys were returned to a drop box or clinic staff and securely stored away from patient records.

The survey asked girls, "Would you be willing to use Planned Parenthood's confidential services for: pregnancy testing and/or counseling, birth control drugs or devices, health exams, HIV testing and/or treatment, testing and/or treatment for other sexually transmitted diseases (STDs)?" Girls indicated whether (yes or no) they would use each confidential service. After stating that "some lawmakers would like to inform parents in writing that their teens are seeking prescribed birth control pills or devices at family planning clinics that receive federal funds," the survey asked: "Would informing your parents cause you to stop using Planned Parenthood services?" The response format was yes or no. If girls responded that they would not stop using all Planned Parenthood services, they were asked to indicate whether they would continue to use specific services: pregnancy testing or counseling, birth control drugs or devices, health examinations, HIV testing or treatment, and testing or treatment for other STDs. For each service, girls responded yes or no. Those who would not stop using all Planned Parenthood services if their parents were informed also indicated whether (yes or no) they would delay testing or treatment for HIV or other STDs.

Participants in the Additional Sample

Additional data were collected in 2001 from 3 Planned Parenthood family planning clinics in Milwaukee, the most densely populated county in Wisconsin. All single, sexually active girls younger than 18 years (n = 256) were asked to complete a confidential, institutional review board-approved survey. Ten percent declined, primarily because of time constraints. A total of 230 sexually active adolescent girls voluntarily completed the survey. The demographic characteristics of girls in the additional sample were virtually identical to those in the statewide sample. The mean age was 16.5 years (SD, 1.24; range, 12–17 years), and 76.1% were white, 15.2% were African American, 5.2% were Hispanic, and 3.5% were Asian.

The same procedure used for the statewide sample was used to survey the additional sample. The survey stated: "Some lawmakers would like to inform parents in writing that their teens are seeking prescribed birth control pills or devices at family planning clinics that receive federal funds." Girls were then asked: "Would informing your parents cause you to stop using Planned Parenthood services?" The response format was yes or no. If girls responded that they would stop using services with parental notification, they then indicated (yes or no) whether they would "stop having sexual intercourse," "use condoms," "use spermicidal foam or gel," "use the rhythm method," have their partner withdraw or "pull out" before ejaculation, or "have unprotected sexual intercourse." Girls were also given the opportunity to indicate *other* and specify what they would do if they stopped using family planning services because of mandatory parental notification.

Statistical Analysis

Descriptive statistics computed for the statewide sample included the percentage of girls who would be willing to use all confidential sexual health care services and the percentage who would stop using sexual health care services if parental notification for prescribed contraceptives were mandated. In addition, calculated in the statewide sample among the girls who would not stop using sexual health care services with parental notification were the percentage who would delay testing or treatment for HIV or other STDs and the percentage who would discontinue using specific (but not all) sexual health services if their parents were informed that they were seeking prescribed contraceptives. The effect of mandatory parental notification on girls' use of sexual health care services by clinic site, race, and age was also analyzed with simultaneous logistic regression analysis to control for possible intercorrelations. χ^2 Analyses were then performed for clinic site, race, and age to follow up the multivariate analysis.

Statistics computed for the additional sample included the percentage who would stop using services with parental notification. Also, the percentage who would stop having sexual intercourse, use condoms, use spermicidal foam or gel, use the rhythm method, have their partner withdraw, or have unprotected sexual intercourse was calculated among those who would stop using sexual health care services with parental notification. For all analyses, SPSS (PSS Inc, Chicago, Ill.) for Windows (version 10.1) was used.

RESULTS

Eighty-six percent (n = 814) of girls in the statewide sample indicated that they would be willing to use all confidential sexual health care services. The remaining 14% (n = 136) of girls indicated that they would be willing to use one confidential sexual health care service or various combinations of confidential sexual health care services but were unwilling to use all services. Forty-seven percent (n = 444) of the sample reported that they would stop using all Planned Parenthood services if their parents were notified that they were seeking prescribed birth control pills or devices. An additional 12% (n = 112) reported that they would change their use of Planned Parenthood services if parental notification became mandatory. Sixty-five girls would delay testing or treatment for HIV or other STDs, and 47 would discontinue using specific sexual health care services. Thirty-six girls would discontinue pregnancy testing, 27 would discontinue STD testing and treatment, 9 would discontinue HIV testing, 9 would discontinue health examinations, and 2 would discontinue using services for birth control. Since some girls indicated that they would discontinue using more than one sexual health care service, the total is 83 rather than 47. The effect of mandatory parental notification on girls' use of sexual health care services was investigated by clinic site, race, and age. An omnibus test of the full model with site, race, and age as predictors indicated that only race and age significantly predicted whether girls would stop using services with parental notification (χ^2_4, 20.8; $P<.001$). For the 2 other main outcome measures, delay in testing or treatment for HIV and other STDs and for discontinuing use of specific (but not all) services, no site, race, or age differences were found (delay: χ^2_4, 4.5; $P = .34$; discontinue: χ^2_4, 3.0; $P = .56$).

Racial differences were investigated by comparing the white girls, the African American girls, and all other girls in the sample combined. There were not enough Hispanic, Native American, and Asian girls in the sample to permit individual comparisons for these groups. Figure 7.1 shows that there were racial differences in whether girls indicated that they would stop using services (χ^2_2, 9.6; $P = .008$). Compared with white girls (χ^2_1, 7.7; $P = .008$) and other

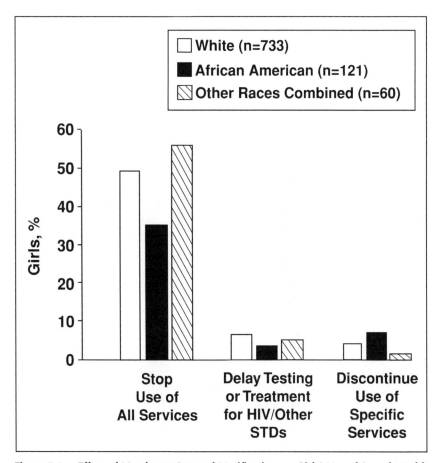

Figure 7.1. Effect of Mandatory Parental Notification on Girls' Use of Sexual Health Care Services by Race

girls of color (χ^2_1, 7.1; P= .008), African American girls were significantly less likely to indicate that they would stop using services if their parents were notified. However, the African American girls did not differ from the other racial subgroups in whether they would delay testing or treatment for HIV or other STDs (χ^2_2, 1.8; $P = .39$) or discontinue using specific (but not all) services (χ^2_2, 0.02; $P = .99$).

Age differences were examined with girls 15 years or younger, 16 years of age, and 17 years of age. Individual comparisons for each age younger than 15 years were impossible because of small sample sizes. As shown in Figure 7.2, the analysis revealed a significant age difference (χ^2_2, 12.4; $P = .002$). Girls 17 years of age were less likely than those 15 years or younger (χ^2_1,

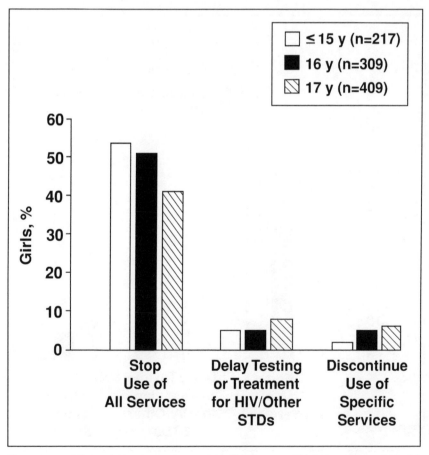

Figure 7.2. Effect of Mandatory Parental Noficiation on Girls' Use of Sexual Health Care Services by Age

10.0; $P = .002$) and 16 years of age (χ_1^2, 7.0; $P = .008$) to indicate that they would stop using sexual health care services if their parents were informed that they were seeking prescribed birth control pills or devices. No differences were found between the age groups in whether they would delay testing or treatment for HIV or other STDs (χ_2^2, 2.3; $P = .31$) or discontinue their use of specific (but not all) services (χ_2^2, 3.6; $P = .16$).

With regard to site, there were no differences between girls seeking sexual health care services at urban clinics vs rural clinics in whether they would stop using services (48.3% urban and 46.9% rural; χ_1^2, 0.2; $P = .64$), delay testing or treatment for HIV or other STDs (6.5% urban and 6.9% rural; χ_1^2, 0.4; $P = .51$), or discontinue their use of specific (but not all) services (6.5% urban and 4.9% rural; χ_1^2, 0.4; $P = .51$) if their parents were informed that they were seeking prescribed birth control pills or devices.

Forty-eight percent (n = 110) of girls in the additional sample indicated that they would stop using services if their parents were notified that they were seeking prescribed birth control pills or devices. Fifty-seven percent indicated that, instead of using services, they would use condoms, 29% indicated that they would have their partner withdraw before ejaculation, 29% indicated that they would have unprotected sexual intercourse, 0% indicated that they would use spermicidal foam or gel, 0% indicated that they would use the rhythm method, and 1% indicated that they would stop having sexual intercourse but would engage in oral sex. (The percentages sum to more than 100% because some girls indicated that they would use more than one method.) Fourteen percent of the girls in this additional sample who said they would use condoms also indicated that they would, at times, have unprotected sexual intercourse or have their partner withdraw before fully ejaculating.

COMMENT

Even though the US courts found that the constitutional right of privacy provides some protection for minors' access to contraceptives (eg, *Carey v Population Services International*, 431 US 678, [1977]), during the past few years numerous federal and state proposals have been introduced that would mandate some form of parental involvement when minors obtain contraceptives. It is important to know what the impact of such proposals would be if they were enacted. The findings of the statewide study show that 59% of the sexually active girls surveyed would stop, delay, or discontinue using specific (but not all) sexual health care services if parental notification were legislated. Previous regional[7] and national[8] surveys found that 36% and 23% of adolescent girls, respectively, would stop using sexual health care services with parental notification. More than 2 decades later, we found that 47% of girls surveyed in Wisconsin would stop using sexual health care services with mandatory parental notification. Consistent with previous reports that 96% to 98% of girls would remain sexually active, 99% of adolescent girls in our additional sample who would stop using sexual health care services with parental notification indicated that they would continue having sexual intercourse despite restricted access to prescribed contraceptives. Given this information, requiring parental notification for obtaining prescribed contraceptives would likely increase unintended pregnancies, abortions, and out-of-wedlock births.

Findings from this statewide investigation also suggest that the effects of parental notification may extend beyond increasing adolescent pregnancies, abortions, and births in that 11% of adolescent girls indicated that if parental notification were required, they would discontinue or delay STD testing and treatment. Every survey question clearly stated that, if legislated, parental notification would occur only for prescribed birth control pills or devices. However, the prospect of parental notification for prescribed contraceptives may have led these girls to question whether HIV and other STD services would be provided in confidence. Consequently, the data suggest that if parental notification were legislated, rates of STDs may increase, not only among adolescent girls who would discontinue using STD tests and treatment, but also among girls for whom STD detection would have occurred during routine gynecological examinations or those related to prescribed contraceptives.

Furthermore, the findings from our additional sample suggest that requiring parental notification for obtaining prescribed contraceptives will not substantially increase consistent condom use. The majority of those who would stop using services with parental notification (56%) indicated that they would at times practice less effective forms of contraception, such as having their partner withdraw or using condoms sporadically. The barriers perceived by adolescent girls (and their sexual partners) to consistently using condoms would have to be addressed before condoms could serve as a feasible substitute for prescribed contraceptives.

Finally, mandatory parental notification was found to be a significant obstacle to girls' use of sexual health care services across all races and ages studied. Almost half (48.8%) of the African American girls and more than half of the white girls (60.3%) and girls classified as other minority (64.2%) would be negatively affected by requiring parental notification. African American girls were less likely to report that they would stop using services with parental notification than were white girls and other minority girls. Greater parental awareness and support of use of contraceptives in African

American daughters and greater openness in regard to sexual matters between African American parents and daughters may account for these findings.[10] Likewise, greater awareness and support of use of contraceptives and greater independence from parents may explain the finding that girls 17 years of age were less likely than the younger girls to report that they would stop using sexual health care services if their parents were informed that they were seeking prescribed contraceptives.[11]

Several limitations of this statewide investigation should be kept in mind. The findings of this investigation are by necessity based on reports of what girls would do if parental notification were required. Girls' actual behavior may differ from their projected behavior. Some girls may have responded in ways they presumed the service providers would want or used their responses to voice their opposition to mandatory parental notification. Although biased responses are always possible in any survey, other research examining the general issue of adolescents' attitudes about parental involvement in their seeking of health care[6] found results similar to ours when the data were collected in schools rather than family planning clinics. Because 45% indicated that they were willing to seek health care for birth control only if their parents did not know and 47% of girls in our statewide survey indicated that they would stop using sexual health services with parental notification, our findings probably are not the result of the family planning clinic context. Although the data were collected from all 33 Planned Parenthood family planning clinics throughout Wisconsin, and all girls who visited clinics during the study period were invited to participate, yielding a high response rate, the percentage of girls who would stop, delay, or discontinue using specific (but not all) sexual health care services with mandatory parental notification might vary from state to state. However, we speculate that the basic conclusion—requiring parental notification for obtaining prescribed contraceptives would impede adolescent girls' use of sexual health care services—would not differ. Finally, we do not have socioeconomic or clinical information on the adolescents to determine which girls might be more affected by mandatory parental notification.

The findings of this statewide investigation support the hypothesis that requiring parental notification for obtaining prescribed contraceptives would impede adolescent girls' use of contraceptive services and their willingness to seek screening and treatment for STDs.

Author Contributions: *Study concept and design:* Reddy, Fleming, Swain. *Acquisition of data:* Reddy, Fleming, Swain. *Analysis and interpretation of data:* Reddy, Fleming. *Drafting of the manuscript:* Reddy, Fleming. *Critical revision of the manuscript for important intellectual content:* Swain.

Statistical expertise: Reddy, Fleming.

Obtained funding: Reddy, Fleming, Swain.

Funding/Support: This work was supported by grants from Planned Parenthood of Wisconsin, Inc, the University of Wisconsin—Milwaukee Center for Urban Initiatives and Research, and the Society for the Psychological Study of Social issues. These funding organizations had no role in the design, conduct, interpretation, or analysis of the study, nor did they review or approve the manuscript.

Disclaimer: The opinions expressed in this chapter do not necessarily reflect those of Planned Parenthood Federation of America.

NOTES

1. 65 *Federal Register* 164.502(g) (2000).

2. Council on Long Range Planning and Development. *AMA Policy Compendium*. Chicago, Ill: American Medical Association; 1990.

3. American College of Obstetricians and Gynecologists. *ACOG Statement of Policy: Confidentiality in Adolescent Health Care*. Washington, DC: American College of Obstetricians and Gynecologists; 1988.

4. Gans J, ed. *Policy Compendium on Confidential Health Services for Adolescents*. Chicago, Ill: American Medical Association; 1993.

5. Council on Scientific Affairs. Confidential health services for adolescents. *JAMA*. 1993;269:1420–1424.

6. Marks A, Malizio J, Hoch J, Brody R, Fisher M. Assessment of health needs and willingness to utilize health care resources of adolescents in a suburban population. *J Pediatr*. 1983;102:456–460.

7. Torres A. Does your mother know? *Fam Plann Perspect*. 1978;10:280–282.

8. Torres A, Forrest JD, Eisman S. Telling parents: clinic policies and adolescents' use of family planning and abortion services. *Fam Plann Perspect*. 1980;12:284–292.

9. Dillman DA. *Mail and Telephone Surveys. The Total Design Method*. New York, NY: John Wiley & Sons; 1978.

10. Raffaelli M, Bogenschneider K, Flood MF. Parent-teen communication about sexual topics. *J Fam Issues*. 1998;19:315–333.

11. Bulcroft RA, Carmody DC, Bulcroft KA. Patterns of parental independence giving to adolescents: variations by race, age, and gender of child. *J Marriage Fam*. 1996;58:866–883.

8

Economic and Health Consequences of Selling a Kidney in India

Madhav Goyal, Ravindra L. Mehta,
Lawrence J. Schneiderman,
and Ashwini R. Sehgal

Context Many countries have a shortage of kidneys available for transplantation. Paying people to donate kidneys is often proposed or justified as a way to benefit recipients by increasing the supply of organs and to benefit donors by improving their economic status. However, whether individuals who sell their kidneys actually benefit from the sale is controversial.

Objective To determine the economic and health effects of selling a kidney.

Design, Setting, and Participants Cross-sectional survey conducted in February 2001 among 305 individuals who had sold a kidney in Chennai, India, an average of 6 years before the survey.

Main Outcome Measures Reasons for selling kidney, amount received from sale, how money was spent, change in economic status, change in health status, advice for others contemplating selling a kidney.

Results Ninety-six percent of participants sold their kidneys to pay off debts. The average amount received was $1070. Most of the money received was spent on debts, food, and clothing. Average family income declined by one third after nephrectomy ($P<.001$), and the number of participants living below the poverty line increased. Three fourths of participants were still in debt at the time of the survey. About 86% of participants reported deterioration in their health status after nephrectomy. Seventy-nine percent would not recommend that others sell a kidney.

Conclusions Among paid donors in India, selling a kidney does not lead to a long-term economic benefit and may be associated with a decline in health. Physicians and policy makers should reexamine the value of using financial incentives to increase the supply of organs for transplantation.

99

Compared with long-term dialysis, renal transplantation generally offers a longer life span and a better quality of life.[1,2] However, nearly every country has a shortage of kidneys for transplantation. In the United States, 50000 individuals are waiting for kidney transplantation, yet only 15000 kidneys are transplanted annually.[3] The shortage is even more severe in developing countries. Despite India's having 4 times the population of the United States, Indian physicians transplant fewer than 4000 kidneys annually, and a number of the organs are received by non-Indians.[4–7]

In the United States, a majority of kidney transplants come from cadaveric donors; eg, brain-dead victims of motor vehicle crashes.[3] In India, no national cadaveric program exists, and virtually all kidneys come from living donors.[8] Because medically suitable living-related donors are often unavailable or unwilling to donate, most transplants are from living-unrelated donors.[4, 9, 10] Moreover, long-term dialysis treatment is federally financed in the United States but not in India. As a result, only a small number of wealthy patients can pay for dialysis treatment in India.[8]

Paying people to donate kidneys is often proposed or justified as a way to increase the supply of organs and help the seller. In the United States, providing financial incentives to families has been proposed as a way to increase the supply of cadaveric organs.[11, 12] Proponents argue that incentives such as paying for funeral expenses will supplement whatever altruistic motivations are already present. However, legal issues as well as concerns about weakening altruism and exploiting poor families have so far prevented these proposals from being implemented.[13, 14]

In India, the purchase of kidneys from living-unrelated donors has occurred for more than a decade.[4, 5, 9, 15, 16] This practice is justified as a way to save the life of patients with no other treatment options and simultaneously help a poor donor overcome extreme poverty.[5, 6, 17–21] Supporters further argue that the seller has the right to choose the fate of his or her kidney and that taking away this option harms the seller financially. They also argue that there is little health risk to the donor from nephrectomy.[21] Critics argue that purchasing kidneys amounts to exploitation of the poor, that the poor do not overcome poverty as a result of the sale, and that this practice prevents a national cadaveric transplant program from being established.[4, 9, 13, 22–32] Critics also view kidney sales not as expressions of individual autonomy but rather as acts of desperation by impoverished individuals.[9] Moneylenders may also be more aggressive in demanding payment from debtors who live in areas where kidneys are sold to pay off debts.[9] Middlemen in particular are criticized as misleading potential donors about what a nephrectomy involves and keeping a large share of the payment. In response to this concern, some clinics purchased organs directly from donors.[5, 6] A 1994 law banned the sale of kidneys and further required that all transplant centers have an authorization committee review potential living-unrelated donations to ensure that donations were made out of altruism and not for commercial reasons.[33, 34] Anecdotal reports suggest that sales of kidneys continue despite this law. Commerce in kidney transplantation also occurs in South America, the Middle East, South Africa, China, and Pakistan.[4, 16, 35]

Table 8.1. Participant Characteristics (N = 305)

	Mean (Median, Range)
Age, y	35 (35, 20–55)
Female, %	71
Education, Y	2.7 (0, 0–12)
Annual family income, $	420 (381, 0–1730)
Income below poverty line, %	71
Time since nephrectomy	6.0y (6.4y, 2wk–19y)
No. of people in household	4.2 (4.0, 1–8)

The value of using financial incentives continues to be controversial despite some qualitative reports indicating that donors who sell their kidney do not benefit and may actually be harmed.[9, 11, 16, 21, 31, 32, 35–41] We sought to contribute to this debate by quantifying the economic and health consequences of selling a kidney among a large sample of sellers.

METHODS

Participants

The study was conducted during February 2001 in Chennai (formerly called Madras), a large city of 6 million people that is the capital of the state of Tamil Nadu in southern India. Adult residents of Chennai were eligible for inclusion if they had sold a kidney. Because most of these transplants are done in secrecy, written records are often unavailable. We therefore relied on snowball sampling, a standard method for contacting difficult-to-reach populations for face-to-face interviews.[42] We used newspaper articles and information provided by transplant professionals to identify neighborhoods of Chennai where sellers resided. A team of 8 Tamil-speaking research assistants identified participants by going door to door in these neighborhoods. They also asked each interviewed participant for names and locations of other people who had sold a kidney. Answers ranged from next-door neighbors to people living in neighborhoods more than 15 km away. Each identified neighborhood was revisited until no more eligible participants were found.

Interview

The research assistants explained the nature of the study, obtained informed written consent, verified that participants had nephrectomy scars, and asked the participants the following questions: why they sold their kidney, whether wanting to help a sick person with kidney disease was a major factor in their decision to sell, why they rather than their spouse had sold, how much money was promised, how much money was received, whether they sold through a middleman or directly to a clinic, how the money was spent, their annual family income currently and before nephrectomy, their health status currently and before nephrectomy, and what advice they would give to others contemplating selling.

Participants also provided their age, sex, education, and date of nephrectomy. Before the interview, participants were given 40 rupees (approximately $0.89) as compensation for their time. They were told that they could keep the money even if they did not want to answer any or all of the questions. Participants were not asked to name particular physicians, middlemen, hospitals, or clinics where the nephrectomy was done. Each interview was recorded on a questionnaire and lasted approximately 20 minutes. The questionnaire was pilot tested on a separate group of 19 participants, and their responses were used to refine the questions. This study was approved by the institutional review board of the University of California, San Diego.

Statistical Analysis

Data are presented by using standard descriptive statistics (mean, median, range, and proportions). We used the paired τ test to compare family income before and after nephrectomy (Stata, version 6; Stata Corp, college Station, Tex). Monetary figures were first adjusted for inflation by using the Indian consumer price index and then converted from rupees to dollars by using the exchange rate at the time of the interview ($1 = 45 rupees).[43–45] The poverty line for Tamil Nadu is $538 a year for an average-sized family.[46]

RESULTS

Participant Characteristics

Of 305 eligible sellers identified, all agreed to participate (Table 8.1). Sixty percent of female participants and 95% of male participants worked as laborers or street vendors. Seventy percent of participants sold their kidneys through a middleman, and 30% sold directly to a clinic.

Reasons for Selling a Kidney

Almost all the participants sold their kidneys to pay off debts (Table 8.2). Food and household expenses, rent, marriage expenses, and medical expenses were the most common sources of these debts. When asked a separate question about wanting to help a sick person with kidney disease, 95% of participants said this was not a major factor in their decision to sell.

Table 8.2.   Reasons for Selling a Kidney*

Reason	No. (%)
Pay off debts	292 (96)
Food/household expenses	160 (55)
Rent	71 (24)
Marriage expenses	65 (22)
Medical expenses	54 (18)
Funeral expenses	23 (8)
Business expenses	23 (8)
Other debts	49 (17)
Future marriage expenses for daughters	10 (3)
Extra cash	4 (1)
Start business	2 (1)
Other reason	3 (1)

*Percentages do not add up to 100% because some participants had more than 1 reason for selling or more than 1 source of debt.

Forty-seven participants noted that their spouse had also sold a kidney. The other 221 married participants (159 female participants and 62 male participants) were asked why they sold rather than their spouse. The most common responses by female participants were that their husbands were the breadwinners (30%) or were ill (28%). The most common responses by male participants were that they sold voluntarily (52%) or that their wives were ill or pregnant (19%). Two female participants stated that they had been forced by their husbands to sell a kidney.

Amount Received from Sale

The amount promised for selling a kidney averaged $1410 (range, $450–$6280), while the amount actually received averaged $1070 (range,

$450–$2660). Both middlemen and clinics promised on average about one third more than they actually paid.

How Money Was Spent

Most of the money received was spent on debts (60%), food and clothing (22%), or marriage (5%). Only 11% was retained as cash equivalents (cash, jewelry, bank deposit, or other investment).

Change in Economic Status

Although the economic status of individuals in Tamil Nadu has improved throughout the last decade, many of the participants reported a worsening of their economic status. Among all participants, the average annual family income declined from $660 at the time of nephrectomy to $420 at the time of the survey, a decrease of one third ($P<.001$). The percentage of participants below the poverty line increased from 54% to 71% ($P<.001$). Of the 292 participants who sold a kidney to pay off debts, 216 (74%) still had debts at the time of the survey.

Change in Health Status

Participants rated their health status before and after nephrectomy by using a 5-point Likert scale ranging from excellent to poor (Table 8.3). Forty participants (13%) reported no decline in their health after nephrectomy, 117 (38%) reported a 1- to 2-point decline, and 147 (48%) reported a 3- to 4-point decline. Of all participants, 50% complained of persistent pain at the nephrectomy site and 33% complained of long-term back pain.

Table 8.3.   Health Status Before and After Nephrectomy

Health Before Nephrectomy	Health After Nephrectomy, No.				
	Excellent	*Very Good*	*Good*	*Fair*	*Poor*
Excellent	11	16	15	58	50
Very good	0	14	16	53	39
Good	0	0	9	10	6
Fair	0	0	1	6	1
Poor	0	0	0	0	0

Advice for Others

Participants were asked what advice they would give someone else with the same reasons they had for selling. Of 264 participants who answered this question, 79% would not recommend selling a kidney, while 21% would.

Time Since Nephrectomy vs Participant Responses

Increased time since nephrectomy was associated with a larger amount received from selling a kidney and a larger decline in economic status. The 47 participants who sold a kidney more than 10 years ago received $1603 compared with $975 for participants who sold within the last 10 years ($P<.001$). Participants who sold more than 10 years ago also reported a 56% decline in annual family income compared with a 29% decline among participants who sold more recently ($P<.001$). There was no relationship between time since nephrectomy and reasons for selling, how the money was spent, changes in health status, and advice for others.

COMMENT

We found widespread evidence of the sale of kidneys by poor people in India despite a legal ban on such sales. In a 1-month period, we were easily able to identify and interview more than 300 individuals who sold a kidney. Selling a kidney did not lead to a long-term economic benefit for the seller and was associated with a decline in health status.

Importance of Results

Our quantitative findings, along with those of previous qualitative studies[9, 16, 31, 32, 34, 35] undercut 5 key assumptions made by supporters of the sale of kidneys. First, although paying people to donate may have increased the supply of organs for transplantation, the financial incentive did not supplement underlying altruistic motivations. Only 5% of participants said wanting to help a sick person was a major factor in their decision to sell. Second, selling a kidney did not help poor donors overcome poverty. Family income actually declined by one third, and most participants were still in debt and living below the poverty line at the time of the survey. Third, regardless of these poor economic outcomes, sellers arguably have a right to make informed decisions about their own bodies. However, most participants would not recommend that others sell a kidney, which suggests that potential donors would be unlikely to sell a kidney if they were better informed of the likely outcomes. Fourth, safeguards such as eliminating middlemen or having an authorization committee did not appear to be effective. Middlemen and clinics paid less than they promised, and the authorization committees did not ensure that donations were motivated by altruism alone. Fifth, nephrectomy was associated with a decline in health status. Previous qualitative reports suggest that a diminished ability to perform physical labor may explain the observed worsening of economic status.[31-35] Persistent pain and decline in health status have not been reported in previous long-term follow-up of volunteer donors in developed countries.[47]

Our findings have important implications for developing and developed countries. In developing countries such as India, potential donors need to be protected from being exploited. At a minimum, protection might involve education about the likely outcomes of selling a kidney. Some have commented that rather than protecting poor people, authorization committees simply provide a cover for illegal cash-for-kidneys deals.[9, 31, 34] Indian legislators should consider modifying the 1994 transplantation act to prevent the sale of organs under such cover. Physicians and policy makers need to work together to develop alternatives for treating renal failure patients. A national cadaveric program is needed, as is an increased emphasis on primary prevention of common diseases that lead to kidney failure. Since paying off debts was the most common reason for selling a kidney, social and economic efforts to reduce or prevent indebtedness are also essential. In developed countries such as the United States, our findings may give pause to efforts to provide financial incentives to encourage donation. In particular, our findings raise concerns about whether providing financial incentives may be viewed by the public as taking advantage of poor families.[14] If perceptions about transplantation are adversely affected, such incentives may actually lead to fewer total donations.

A majority of donors were women. Given the often weak position of women in Indian society, the voluntary nature of some donations is questionable.[48] In fact, 2 participants said that their husbands forced them to donate. Because the interviews were generally conducted with other family members present, other participants may have been reluctant to mention being forced to donate. In the United States, women are also more likely to be donors than men[49], but in both countries, men are more likely to receive transplants.[3, 50]

Limitations

Several alternative interpretations of our results must be considered. First, our findings may simply represent general declines in the economic and health status of poor people in India and not declines linked to the sale of a kidney. However, although data on self-reported health status are lacking, per capita income for Tamil Nadu has increased by 10% over the last 5 years and by 37% over the last 10 years after adjustment for inflation.[51, 52] Additionally, the proportion of people living below the poverty line has declined by more than 50% since 1988.[51–54]

Second, participants may have overestimated their economic and health status before nephrectomy. Among poor people in India, virtually all financial transactions are conducted in cash, and bank accounts are nonexistent. As a result, there are no written financial records that can be used to independently verify participant responses.[9] Written medical records are similarly lacking. However, participant responses to questions about their current economic and health status would not be susceptible to a similar recall bias. According to these responses, we can still conclude that participants have debt, live in poverty, have a fair to poor health status, and would not recommend that others sell a kidney.

Third, the adverse experiences of our participants may not represent those of other sellers. For example, some sellers may have obtained such a large economic benefit that they moved out of the low-income neighborhoods that were the focus of our study. However, no interviewed participant mentioned such individuals when asked for locations of other people who had sold a kidney. In addition, our findings are consistent with those of other qualitative reports.[9, 16, 31, 32] These alternative interpretations could be further addressed in studies involving a comparison group, prospective follow-up, independently verified measures of economic and health status, and additional geographic areas. Other topics not explored in this study include the nature of any relationship between participants and recipients, the reasons sellers failed to realize an economic benefit, the reasons their health deteriorated, the reasons the amount received for selling has declined, and the perspectives and roles of recipients, transplant surgeons, middlemen, and donors' families.

CONCLUSION

The sale of kidneys by poor people in India does not lead to a tangible benefit for the seller. The value of paying for donations must be reexamined in light of these findings. Although patients with kidney failure deserve access to optimal treatment, such treatment should not be based on the exploitation of poor people.

Author Contributions: *Study concept and design*: Goyal, Mehta, Sehgal. *Acquisition of data:* Goyal. *Analysis and interpretation of data:* Goyal, Schneiderman, Sehgal. *Drafting of the manuscript:* Goyal, Mehta, Sehgal. *Critical revision of the manuscript for important intellectual content:* Goyal, Mehta, Schneiderman, Sehgal. *Statistical expertise:* Goyal, Sehgal. *Administrative, technical, or material support:* Mehta. *Study supervision:* Sehgal.

Acknowledgment: We are grateful for the assistance of transplant professionals who helped us locate sellers, for the hard work of the research assistants, and for the willingness of the participants to share their experiences with us. We also appreciate the input of students and lecturers in the course Activism and Medicine at Case Western Reserve University.

NOTES

1. Wolfe RA, Ashby VB, Milford EL, et al. Comparison of mortality in all patients on dialysis, patients on dialysis awaiting transplantation, and recipients of a first cadaveric transplant. *N Engl J Med*. 1999;341:1725–1730.

2. Evans RW, Manninen DL, Garrison LP Jr, et al. The quality of life of patients with end-stage renal disease. *N Engl J Med*, 1985;312:553–559.

3. United Network for Organ Sharing. US facts about transplantation. Available at: http://www.unos.org /frame_Default.asp?Category=Newsdata. Accessibility verified August 9, 2002.

4. Chugh KS, Jha V. Commerce in transplantation in third world countries. *Kidney Int*. 1996;49:1181–1186.

5. Reddy KC, Thiagrajan CAA, Shunmugasundaram D, et al. Unconventional renal transplantation in India. *Transplant Proc*. 1990;22:910–911.

6. Thiagrajan CM, Reddy KC, Shunmugasundaram D, et al. The practice of unconventional renal transplantation (UCRT) at a single center in India. *Transplant Proc*. 1990;22:912–914.

7. Chengappa R. The organs bazaar. *India Today*. July 31, 1990:60–67.

8. Kher V. End-stage renal disease in developing countries. *Kidney Int*. 2002;62:350–362.

9. Cohen L. Where it hurts: Indian material for an ethics of organ transplantation. *Daedalus*. 1999;128:135–165.

10. Marshall PA, Daar AS. Cultural and psychological dimensions of human organ transplantation. *Ann Transplant* 1998;3:7–11.

11. Delmonico FL, Arnold R, Scheper-Hughes N, Siminoff LA, Kahn J, Youngner SJ. Ethical incentives—not payment—for organ donation. *N Engl J Med*. 2002; 346:2002–2005.

12. Josefson D. AMA considers whether to pay for donation of organs. *BMJ*. 2002;324:1541.

13. Peters TG. Life or death: the issue of payment in cadaveric organ donation. *JAMA*. 1991;265:1302–1305.

14. Sehgal A, LeBeau S, Youngner S. Dialysis patient attitudes toward financial incentives for kidney donation. *Am J Kidney Dis*. 1997;29:410–418.

15. Salahudeen AK, Woods HF, Pingle A, et al. High mortality among recipients of bought living-unrelated donor kidneys. *Lancet*. 1990;336:725–728.

16. Scheper-Hughes N. The global traffic in human organs. *Curr Anthropol*. 2000;41:192–224.

17. Daar AS. Rewarded gifting. *Transplant Proc*. 1992; 24:2207–2211.

18. Radcliffe-Richards J. From him that hath not. In: Land W. Dossetor JB, eds. *Organ Replacement Therapy: Ethics, Justice and Commerce*. Berlin, Germany: Springer-Verlag;1991:191.

19. Patel CT. Live renal donation: a viewpoint. *Transplant Proc*. 1988;20(suppl 1): 1068.

20. Reddy KC. Organ donation for consideration: an Indian viewpoint. In: Land W, Dossetor JB, eds. *Organ Replacement Therapy., Ethics, Justice and Commerce*. Berlin, Germany: Springer-Verlag; 1991:173– 180.

21. Kennedy I, Sells RA, Daar AS, et al. The case for "presumed consent" in organ donation. *Lancet*. 1998;351:1650–1652.

22. Abouna GM, Kumar MSA, Samhan M, Dadah SK, John P, Sabawi NM. Commercialization in human organs: a Middle Eastern perspective. *Transplant Proc*. 1990;22:918–921.

23. Al-Khader AA, Al-Sulaiman M, Dhar JM. Living non-related kidney transplantation in Bombay [letter]. *Lancet*. 1990;336:1002.

24. The Council of the Transplantation Society. Commercialization in transplantation: the problems and some guidelines for practice. *Lancet*. 1985;2:715–716.

25. Medawar P, Dausset J, Snell G. Markets in kidneys [letter]. *Lancet*. 1984;2:1344.

26. Mani MK. Renal transplantation in India. *Transplant Proc*. 1992; 24:1828–1829.

27. Colabawalla BN. High mortality among recipients of bought living-unrelated donor kidneys [letter]. *Lancet*. 1990;336:1194.

28. Pellegrino ED. Families' self-interest and the cadaver's organs: what price consent? *JAMA*. 1991; 265:1305–1306.

29. Murray TH. Con: the moral repugnance of rewarded gifting. *Transplant Immunt Lett*. 1992;8:5–7.

30. Caplan AL, Van Buren CT, Tilney NL. Financial compensation for cadaver organ donation: good idea or anathema. *Transplant Proc*. 1993;25:2740–2742.

31. Zargooshi J. Iranian kidney donors: motivations and relations with recipients. *J Urol*. 2001;165:386–392.

32. Zargooshi J. Quality of life of Iranian kidney "donors" *J Urol*. 2001;166: 1790–1799.

33. Frontline. Kidneys still for sale. Available at: http: //www.flonnet.com/fl1425/ 14250640.htm. Accessibility verified August 9, 2002.

34. Frontline. Karnataka's unabating kidney trade. Available at: http://www.frc .ntlineonnet.com/ktrade.htm. Accessibility verified August 9, 2002.

35. Finkel M. Complications. *New York Times Magazine*. May 27, 2001:26.

36. Velasco N. Organ donation and kidney sales [letter]. *Lancet*. 1998;352:483.

37. Drukker A. Organ donation and kidney sales [letter]. *Lancet*. 1998;352: 483–484.

38. Lyon S. Organ donation and kidney sales [letter]. *Lancet*. 1998;352:484.

39. Oreopoulos DG. Organ donation and kidney sales [letter]. *Lancet*. 1998;352:484.

40. Khan IH. Organ donation and kidney sales [letter]. *Lancet*. 1998;352:484.

41. Soper C. Organ donation and kidney sales [letter]. *Lancet*. 1998;352:484–485.

42. Lopes CS, Rodrigues LC, Sichieri R. The lack of selection bias in a snowball sampled case-control study on drug abuse. *Int J Epidemiol*. 1996;25:1267–1270.

43. Labour Bureau, Government of India. Index numbers. Available at: http://chd.nic.in/labour/indtab.html. Accessibility verified August 12, 2002.

44. *Yearbook of Labour Statistics 2000*. 59th ed. Geneva, Switzerland: International Labour Office; 2000.

45. *Statistical Yearbook 1992.* 39th ed. New York, NY: United Nations Publication; 1994:341.

46. Planning Commission, Government of India. Poverty estimates for 1999–2000. Available at: http://planningcommission.nic.in/prfebt.htm. Accessibility verified August 9, 2002.

47. Saran R, Marshall SM, Madsen R, Keavey P, Tapson JS. Long-term follow-up of kidney donors: a longitudinal study. *Nephrol Dial Transplant.* 1997;12:1615–1621.

48. Dreze J, Sen A. India: *Economic Development and Social Opportunity.* New York, NY: Oxford University Press; 1995:109–178.

49. Bloembergen WE, Port FK, Mauger EA, Briggs JP, Leichtman AB. Gender discrepancies in living related renal transplant donors and recipients. *J Am Soc Nephrol.* 1996;7:1139–1144.

50. Jha V, Muthukumar T, Kohli HS, Sud K, Gupta KL, Sakhuja V. Impact of cyclosporine withdrawal on living related renal transplants: a single-center experience. *Am J Kidney Dis.* 2001;37:119–124.

51. *India: Reducing Poverty, Accelerating Development A World Bank Country Study.* Oxford, England: Oxford University Press; 2000.

52. State Government of Tamil Nadu, Tamil Nadu at a glance: 2000. Available at: http://www-tn.gov.in /deptst/glance.htm. Accessibility verified August 9, 2002.

53. United Nations Population Fund for United Nations System in India. *India: Towards Population and Development Goals.* Oxford, England: Oxford University Press: 1997.

54. Planning Commission, Government of India. Poverty estimates for 1999–2000. Available at: http: //www.planningcommission.nic.in/ar_table2. htm. Accessibility verified August 9, 2002.

9

Scholarly Watchdogs for an Ethical Netherworld

Peter Monaghan

Among the more mind-boggling developments in modern life, surely, is the possibility of selling one's kidney—let alone having it stolen from one's body during an operation.

Advances in transplant surgery have fostered not only the legal trade of organs and tissues, but also an illegal international trade, in which brokers and transplant clinics cheaply obtain the kidneys—and heart valves, skin, eyes, and pineal glands—of poor people around the world.

Increasingly, body parts are harvested without consent from the families of the dead, and sometimes from the living. Commonly, however, poverty drives people to sell their organs—kidneys, most often, but in the future, hands? Feet?

"Call it neocannibalism—the notion that we can eye each other greedily as a source of spare body parts," says Nancy Scheper-Hughes, a professor of anthropology at the University of California at Berkeley.

The seemingly unstoppable, illegal trafficking of organs has been denounced by numerous international medical and human-rights groups. In many countries, however, so-called body mafias of organ brokers have proved as resourceful as runners of any other contraband.

Ms. Scheper-Hughes is the driving force behind Organs Watch, a research unit set up here last fall that generates and gathers research on organ trafficking. Its associates also assess social and ethical dilemmas raised by transplant medicine.

"Transplant surgery has entered a global market," says Ms. Scheper-Hughes, who heads Berkeley's doctoral program in medical anthropology. "In the organs-trade business, abuses creep in before you know it."

Her interest in the pitfalls of organ transplantation is shared by a growing number of others. . . . About 450 researchers and human-rights workers attended an Organs Watch conference here to discuss various forms of "commodification of human bodies." Anthropologists, human-rights activists, physicians, and medical ethicists are monitoring the trade, and struggling to define the line between ethical and exploitative organ harvesting.

Most of the activities Ms. Scheper-Hughes and her colleagues track involve the abuse of vulnerable people. Organs, whether legally or illegally obtained, flow predominantly from poor to rich, women to men, nonwhite to white.

INTERNATIONAL ABUSES

In South Africa, during the end of the apartheid era, Ms. Scheper-Hughes saw cadavers of poor victims of murder and other violence stripped of skin, eyes, and heart valves without family consent, for use in hospitals in that country and abroad.

In China, authorities harvest organs from the bodies of executed prisoners. Amnesty International and other human-rights groups allege that China has expanded the number and variety of capital crimes to increase organ supply and generate more export income, and that executions are often timed to meet with the needs of paying organ recipients. China has steadfastly denied all those allegations.

In Israel, Ms. Scheper-Hughes recently tracked an organ-brokering doctor who, after being caught sending Israeli Arabs into the West Bank to recruit Palestinians willing to sell organs intended for Israeli buyers, has switched to "kidney tourism" in Turkey, the Middle East, and Eastern Europe.

Organs Watch stems from the work of an international committee convened in 1994 by the Soros Foundation's Open Society Institute: The Bellagio Task Force on Securing Bodily Integrity for the Socially Disadvantaged in Transplant Surgery. Ms. Scheper-Hughes was one of 14 members of the group which also included transplant surgeons, organ-procurement specialists, and human-rights activists. When the committee disbanded in 1996, she obtained grants from the institute and from Berkeley to continue the research and help operate Organs Watch, which she runs with Lawrence Cohen, another professor of anthropology here. Researchers at Organs Watch have done studies in Argentina, Brazil, Cuba, India, Israel, South Africa, and Turkey, among other countries.

Their findings paint a morbid picture. In addition to illegal tissue removal from corpses, documented abuses include:

- The outright theft of organs during operations.
- The granting of release time to prisoners who "donate" organs.
- Corruption of organ waiting lists, and the pressuring by employers of, for example, domestic workers, to trade a kidney in return for job security.
- The involvement of organized-crime rings in the trade of tissues taken from cadavers at hospitals and morgues, in league with staff and ambulance drivers.

Other abuses Ms. Scheper-Hughes has witnessed suggest unimaginable actions. During the 1980's, in Argentina and Brazil morgues, she saw bodies of dead kidnap victims with missing organs. Such deaths fueled public fears that police and soldiers were murdering street children and other civilians to supply organs for officials of the military dictatorships and members of other élite groups.

Ms. Scheper-Hughes says the evidence is inconclusive. But it seems people in high places didn't want her digging up any more of it. During a recent visit to Brazil, where she has performed fieldwork since 1964, Ms. Scheper-Hughes fled after being informed that a hit man hired by a judge involved in organ trafficking was trailing her. "I took it seriously enough that I just left," she says. "This is big business."

SKEPTICAL PEERS

Colleagues have questioned what an anthropologist is doing studying organ trafficking. In the April issue of *Current Anthropology*, for example, Mac Marshall, a professor of anthropology at the University of Iowa, objected that Ms. Scheper-Hughes's approach involved too little ethnography, and depended too much on published reports and journalistic accounts.

She acknowledged in a published response that the urgent task of documenting abuses does lead to "odd juxtapositions of ethnography, fact-finding, documentation/ surveillance, photojournalism, and human-rights advocacy." But she defended her partial reliance on the work of investigative journalists, with whom she has often worked—including for example, some from *60 Minutes*.

"Surely," she wrote, "the time for assumptions of professional superiority is over."

Not all of the questionable traffic in organs happens in foreign countries. Organs have been shipped illegally from Third World countries to at least a few American hospitals and tissue banks. Using the rhetoric of "you can save a life," tissue banks have pressured families to donate bodies of deceased relatives, only to turn around and sell them to biotech companies for use in commercial products. At the University of California at Irvine last year, Christopher C. Brown, the head of the medical school's willed-body program, was dismissed for allegedly selling donated bodies to private companies for car-crash testing and dissection classes for undergraduate premed students. The case is still under investigation.

Last year, a kidney was offered for sale on the eBay Internet auction site. Bidding raced to $5.7million before company officials pulled it because it was contrary to company policy and federal law.

But focusing on such episodes, as Ms. Scheper-Hughes does, is an approach not all transplant researchers share, and some disapprove. The chairman of the Bellagio group, David J. Rothman, who directs the Center for the Study of Society and Medicine at Columbia University, and his wife, Sheila M. Rothman, a professor of public health at Columbia, once collaborated with Ms. Scheper-Hughes, but no longer do.

"We're really looking to promote trust, and not to raise scandals," says Ms. Rothman. "That's where we differ a great deal from the Berkeley group." Transplantation is "a very, very important life-saving procedure," she says.

Her research at dialysis centers shows that patients who need kidney transplants must increasingly consider live donors—generally, in this country, relatives—because donations of cadaveric organs are flat, and transplant waiting lists are long.

"None of this is to imply that sale is going on," she says. And, yes, it is essential to ensure that sales do not crop up "as we move into new territory." But scandals, she suggests, can be "moments for understanding," a way, if handled properly to bring about legal protections.

That may be, says Ms. Scheper-Hughes, but fears about organ donation will remain justified "until there's a massive owning up by the transplant world and the harvesting world and the biotech companies that there has been a real shift towards commercialization" and until informed-consent forms ask: "'Do you object if your loved one's or your own body part may be used in commercial products?'"

GLOBAL QUESTIONS

Beyond the debates over ethics, Ms. Scheper-Hughes says, she also wishes to understand "larger anthropological issues." Some anthropologists argue for a basic continuity between organ trafficking and earlier practices. Ruth Richardson, an honorary research fellow at University College London, suggests in an essay in *Organ Transplantation: Meanings and Realities* (University of Wisconsin Press, 1996) that there is little difference between governments' presuming blanket consent to organ donations upon death—a practice growing in Europe and elsewhere—and the use of executed criminals for dissection practice in 17th-century England.

Ms. Scheper-Hughes agrees, but adds, "What is new, I think, is the globalization of medical practice. The idea that you can extend life through getting someone else's organ is, I think, a quantum leap." She is writing a book tentatively titled *The End(s) of the Body: Human Sacrifice in the Global Age.* What is emerging, she argues, is a completely new way of thinking about the body as a collection of redundancies: People think, "I have two kidneys (or eyes, or ears); I need only one."

For an anthropologist, organ donation touches on many issues of interest, including human relations, values, gift-giving, and commodification of bodies. "Those are the most social of practices," notes Ms. Scheper-Hughes.

Her colleague Mr. Cohen examines just those issues in his work in a part of southern India popularly known as "the kidney belt." His research has taken him to some weird places. This summer, he visited a sweltering "organs motel" fashioned from a residence in a middle-class apartment building in Madras, situated between two private hospitals on a main road. "There were about 10 people lounging on mats on the floor, waiting to sell their kidneys, waiting until someone came with a match," he recalls.

That such sales commonly occur is well documented—by, for example, Patricia Marshall, an associate professor of medical humanities at Loyola University of Chicago. Since the 1970's, southern Indian peasants and slum dwellers, often women, have sold their kidneys—usually for $1,000 to $2,000—to brokers who then sell them to hospitals that contract with wealthy recipients, mostly Indians, Sri Lankans, Bangladeshis, and citizens of Gulf states.

Mr. Cohen's interest in the subject arose several years ago. While preparing a book on old age in India, he began to hear talk of kidney sales among the urban poor. It differed from hushed rumors of organ theft in Latin America, in that it arose in everyday conversation—often in connection with talk of dowries, a tradition then in revival.

But in 1996, he witnessed a regular "kidney panic."

"People were convinced there was a gang of people stealing kids for kidneys," he says. Most likely, he reasons, organ-theft rumors hold little truth. After all, why run the risk of stealing kidneys when they are so openly, though illegally, sold?

The rumors may have been fueled by the fact that Indian clinics, since the liberalization of medical services in the 1980's, were in stiff competition with one another. High numbers of transplant operations were a badge of modernity. Until there was a stable supply of legally obtained organs, "it's quite possible that certain sorts of extraordinary malfeasance could occur," he says.

"Working with Nancy has taught me that for every 10 stories you're convinced couldn't be true, there's one that is true, and is astoundingly true."

Ethical considerations around such practices are not simple, he suggests.
On one side is the insistence on the body's integrity. On the other is the argument that people should have the right to do as they wish with their own bodies, and that to prevent them from selling their organ may push them into
other, more awful choices.

KIDNEYS OR KIDS?

Mr. Cohen discovered in India that successful clinics had learned "to stand
behind the contemporary language of utilitarian ethics." One clinic official
pulled out articles by Janet Radcliffe-Richards, a British philosopher who in
1998 published one titled "The Case for Allowing Kidney Sales," in the
British medical journal, *The Lancet.* Among its arguments was that if people
are kept from selling their kidneys, they may feel forced, say, to sell their children into sex work or bonded labor.

That position is shared by some members of the Bellagio committee.
Among the recommendations of the group was one to regulate organ sales,
rather than attempt to prohibit them.

Ms. Scheper-Hughes says talk of "informed choice" has little relevance
when the poor of Calcutta or Brazilian shanty-towns opt to sell a kidney:
Their decisions are "anything but free and autonomous."

Some of the letters and e-mails that flood into Organs Watch are almost
unimaginable. Eager would-be sellers of organs, after logging onto the organization's Internet site (http://sunsite.berkeley.edu/biotech/organswatch), apparently are confused about the center's work.

Art, "22 years old and completely healthy" and a native speaker of Span-
ish, writes, "My economic situation is not the best, for which if someone of
his patient is interested in obtaining the kidney that I am giving and he has the
economic power for make this possible, I mean, enough money for me and
my family, then, we'll be speaking of a transplante immediate."

10

Clinical and Organizational Factors Associated with Feeding Tube Use among Nursing Home Residents with Advanced Cognitive Impairment

Susan L. Mitchell, Joan M. Teno, Jason Roy,
Glen Kabumoto, and Vincent Mor

ABSTRACT

Context Empiric data and expert opinion suggest that use of feeding tubes is not beneficial for older persons with advanced dementia. Previous research has shown a 10–fold variation in this practice across the United States.

Objective To identify the facility and resident characteristics associated with feeding use among US nursing homes residents with severe cognitive impairment.

Design, Setting, and Participants Cross-sectional study of all residents with advanced cognitive impairment who had Minimum Data Set assessments within 60 days of April (N = 186 835) and who resided in Medicare- or Medicaid-certified US nursing homes.

Main Outcomes Measures Facility and resident characteristics described in the 1999 On-line Survey and Certification of Automated Records and the 1999 Minimum Data Set. Multivariate analysis using generalized estimating equations determined the facility and resident factors independently associated with feeding tube use.

Results Thirty-four percent of residents with advanced cognitive impairment had feeding tubes (N=63 101). Resident characteristics associated with a greater likelihood of feeding tube use included younger age, nonwhite race, male sex, divorced marital status, lack of advance directives, a recent decline in functional status, and no diagnosis of Alzheimer disease. Controlling for these patient factors, residents living in facilities that were for profit (adjusted odds ratio [OR], 1.09; 95% confidence interval [CI], 1.06–1.12); located in an urban area [OR], 1.14; 95% CI, 1.11–1.16); having more than 100 beds (OR, 1.04; 95% CI, 1.01–1.07); and lacking a special dementia care unit (OR, 1.11; 95% CI, 1.07–1.15) had a higher likelihood of having a feeding tube. Additionally, feeding tube use was more likely among residents living in facilities that had a smaller proportion of residents with do-not-resuscitate orders, had a higher prevalence of nonwhite residents, and lacked a nurse practitioner or physician assistant on staff.

Conclusions More than one third of severely cognitively impaired residents in US nursing homes have feeding tubes. Feeding tube use is independently associated with both the residents' clinical characteristics and the nursing homes' fiscal, organizational, and demographic features.

INTRODUCTION

A growing proportion of the approximately 4 million older US adults with Alzheimer disease or other dementias are now surviving to the advanced stages of their illness. Eating and swallowing problems typically develop during the terminal stages of dementias. Whether to initiate feeding tube use or to focus on comfort is one of the most challenging dilemmas facing families, clinicians, and institutions caring for these patients.[1–2]

The widespread use of feeding tubes among older persons with advanced cognitive impairment in the United States[3] is concerning amid growing empirical data and expert opinion indicating that feeding tube use has no demonstrable health benefits in this population and may be associated with increased risks and discomfort.[1–2] For physician and/or institution practice to change, the factors that influence feeding tube use among individuals with advanced cognitive impairment must be understood. These influences may include the clinical characteristics of the patient, the quality of the shared decision-making process, cultural attitudes toward death and dying, and organizational features specific to the health care environment in which the patient is receiving care.

The prevalence of feeding tube use varies considerably among nursing home residents with advanced dementia who are living in different facilities[4], states[3, 5] and countries.[6] These observations suggest that broader influences, which are external to the patient, are important determinants of this practice. A recent study found a 10–fold variation in feeding tube use across the United States.[3] However, only state differences in the use of do-not-resuscitate (DNR) orders were found to be associated with the practice, whereas regional laws governing hydration and state Medicaid reimbursement policies were not. Therefore, additional research is needed to understand the substantial variation in feeding tube use.

To date, investigations attempting to identify factors associated with feeding tube use in this population have examined individual patient variables[5, 7–9] or nursing home characteristics, such as size, location, case-mix, staffing, and fiscal organization, separately.[4] However, these factors do not operate independently. To address this limitation, we linked 2 large national databases; 1 containing administrative, fiscal, and aggregated clinical information on all licensed US nursing homes[10] and the second containing detailed demographic, functional, and clinical data about the residents living in these facilities.[11] Our objective was to examine how patient factors and facility characteristics independently influence feeding tube use among severely cognitively impaired older persons residing in US nursing homes.

METHODS

Study Population

The study population was characterized using data from the 1999 National Repository Resident Assessment Instrument Minimum Data Set (MDS).[11] Data were derived from the MDS assessments completed within 60 days of April 1, 1999, on nursing home residents living in all Medicare- or Medicaid-certified US facilities during that period. Full MDS assessments are completed within 2 weeks of nursing home admission, annually, and whenever there is a significant change in status. Briefer assessments are completed on a quarterly basis. Only full MDS assessments were analyzed in this study. We excluded residents whose reason for their MDS assessment was nursing home admission. The CMDS data for the remaining individuals represented random periods in their nursing home stay.

Residents were included in the study sample if they had advanced cognitive impairment as defined by a cognitive performance score (CPS) of six.[12–13] The CPS uses 5 MDS variables to group residents into 7 hierarchical cognitive performance categories. These categories include 0 = intact; 1 = borderline intact; 2 = mild impairment; 3 = moderate impairment; 4 = moderately severe impairment; 5 = severe impairment; and 6 = very severe impairment with eating problems. Residents identified as comatose were excluded. The MDS was used to determine feeding tube use among residents. The MDS does not distinguish between different types of feeding tubes.

Resident characteristics that were potentially associated with the use of feeding tubes were selected from the data set a priori.[5, 7–9] These characteristics included age; sex; race or ethnicity; marital status; advance directives ((DNR order, living will, and durable power of attorney for health care); diagnosis of Alzheimer disease, stroke, or cancer; and deterioration in the ability to perform activities of daily living activities during the past 90 days (based on a specific MDS variable). Age was grouped in 5–year ranges (<65, 65–69, 70–74, 75–79, 80–84, 85–89, and >90 years, which was the referent category). Race or ethnicity was categorized as American Indian/Alaska Native, Asian/Pacific Islander, black (not of Hispanic origin), Hispanic, and white (not of Hispanic origin), which was the referent category. Marital status was categorized as married, which was the referent category, never married, separated, widowed, or divorced.

Facility Characteristics

Facility characteristics were obtained from the MDS and the On-line Survey Certification of Automated Records (OSCAR) data sets from 1999.[10] OSCAR is a national database of information collected annually as part of the nursing home survey and recertification process; it contains data on facility demographics and corporate structure, staffing, and aggregated patient data. Facility characteristics that may be associated with the use of feeding tubes among residents with advanced cognitive impairment were selected a priori.[4,9] All licensed nursing homes in the United States were included in the analysis (N=15 135).

Facility variables were size (dichotomized at 100 beds, the median), urban vs rural location, and fiscal characteristics and ownership including chain membership, profit status, and whether Medicaid was the primary payer for 80% or more of the beds in the facility. We also determined whether the facility had a special care unit for dementia.

The level of staffing for nurses and certified nursing assistants was defined as the number of full-time (35 h/wk) equivalents per bed. These variables were categorized as less than 0.20 full-time equivalents, which was the referent category, 0.21–0.40, 0.41–0.60, or higher than 0.60. Facilities were dichotomized based on whether they had a full-time speech therapist employed on staff (at least 35 h/wk) and a nurse practitioner or physician assistant on staff who performed physician-delegated services.

The MDS data were used to create several aggregated patient variables based on all residents in the facility—not just those in the study sample—to describe specific nursing home characteristics that were unavailable in the OSCAR data set. The proportion of residents in each facility with a DNR order was grouped as less than 10%, 11%-20%, 21%-40%, 41%-60%, 61%-80%, and higher than 80%, which was the referent category. The racial or ethnic makeup of the facility was defined as the percentage of nonwhite residents and categorized as 0%, which was the referent category, 0.1%-5.0%,

5.1% and higher than 10%. The proportion of residents receiving intravenous therapy was included to reflect the use of other invasive therapies by the facility and grouped as 0%, 0.1%-1.0%, 1.1%-5.0%, 5.1%-10.0%, and higher than 10.0%, which was the referent category. Finally, certain nursing homes may attract tube-fed patients. To adjust for this factor, we determined the proportion of residents with severe cognitive impairment admitted to each facility with feeding tubes in 1999 and categorized this variable as less than 1.0%, which was the referent category, 1.0%-5.0%, 5.1%-10.0%, and higher than 10.%.

Analysis

The dependent variable was whether a resident with advanced cognitive impairment had a feeding tube. As such, the resident was the unit of analysis. The independent variables were grouped as characteristic of individual residents and characteristics of the facilities in which the residents with advanced dementia lived. Descriptive statistics were used to present the proportion of tube-fed and nontube-fed residents with each independent variable.

Multivariate analysis of the dichotomous outcome (the presence of a feeding tube) was performed using logistic regression models with the generalized estimating equation approach in SAS PROC GEN MOD.[14] The generalized estimating equation method adjusts for the correlation among patients residing in the same nursing facility. All the aforementioned resident and facility characteristics were included as independent variables and entered into the multivariate analysis. Therefore, the final logistic regression model adjusts for all resident and facility characteristics. Adjusted odds ratios (ORs) and 95% confidence intervals (CIs) were derived from these analyses. When the outcome is not a rare event, as in this study, the OR may overestimate the risk ratio. Therefore, the method by Zhang and Yu[15] was used to correlate all the ORs.

Variability in Feeding-Tube Practice

To describe the variability in feeding-tube practice in nursing homes within and among states, the proportion of residents with advanced cognitive impairment who had feeding tubes was determined and categorized based on terciles of less than 16%, 16%-40%, and greater than 40%. The percentage of nursing homes in each category was determined for all states. The states were also ranked from those with greatest percentage of facilities in the highest tercile (>40%) to those with the fewest nursing homes in that category. In addition, the proportion of tube-fed residents in each state was determined.

RESULTS

A total of 186 835 nursing home residents in this nationwide sample had a CPS score of 6 (very severe impairment with eating problems); of these, 33.8% (n = 63 101) had feeding tubes. The prevalence of feeding tube use among residents in the other CPS categories is 6965 (2.0%) of 356 761 for a CPS score of 0 (intact); 6012 (3.1%) of 190 731 for a CPS score of 1 (borderline intact); 6454 (3.2%) of 201 777 for a CPS score of 2 (mild impairment); 18 128 (4.5%) of 400 402 for a CPS score of 3 (moderate impairment); 15 141 (11.9%) of 127 275 for a CPS score of 4 (moderately severe impairment); and 2619 (1.9%) of 135 964 for a CPS score of 5 (severe impairment). Table 10.1 describes the facility and clinical characteristics of the residents. Table 10.2 presents the results of multivariate analysis, adjusting for all resident and facility characteristics.

Table 10.1.   Resident and Facility Characteristics of Tube-Fed Residents With Advanced Cognitive Impairment in US Nursing Homes

Characteristic	No. of Residents With Characteristic	No. (%) of Residents With Feeding Tubes Characteristic Present	Characteristic Absent
Resident characteristics (N = 186 835)			
Age, y			
<65	14987	8115 (54)	54986 (32)
65–69	7072	3064 (43)	60037 (33)
70–74	14100	5535 (39)	57566 (33)
75–79	26605	9522 (36)	53579 (33)
80–84	38013	12316 (32)	50785 (34)
85–90	41633	12818 (31)	50283 (35)
≥90	44425	11731 (26)	51370 (36)
Men	44446	18806 (42)	44 295 (31)
Race or ethnicity			
White (not of Hispanic origin)	151597	42455 (28)	20646 (59)
American Indian/Alaska Native	860	343 (40)	62758 (34)
Hispanic	5427	2873 (53)	60228 (33)
Black (not of Hispanic origin)	26653	16028 (60)	47073 (29)
Asian/Pacific Islander	2298	1402 (61)	61699 (33)
Marital status			
Married	48415	17015 (35)	46086 (33)
Never married	21588	9194 (43)	53907 (33)
Widowed	104214	31417 (30)	31684 (38)
Separated	2349	1125 (48)	61976 (34)
Divorced	10269	4350 (42)	58751 (33)

continued

Table 10.1. *(continued)*

Characteristic	No. of Residents With Characteristic	No. (%) of Residents With Feeding Tubes	
		Characteristic Present	Characteristic Absent
Absent			
Do-not-resuscitate order	66537	29203 (44)	33898 (28)
Durable power of attorney for health care	140692	52741 (37)	10360 (22)
Living will	155001	56145 (36)	6956 (22)
Diagnosis of Alzheimer disease	140390	52790 (38)	10311 (22)
Diagnosis of cancer	176522	59720 (34)	3381 (33)
Present			
Diagnosis of stroke	53184	27349 (51)	35752 (27)
Recent decline in functional status	35776	12703 (36)	50398 (33)
Facility Characteristics (N = 15135)			
No dementia special care unit	147764	53012 (36)	10089 (26)
Urban location	135227	49337 (36)	13764 (27)
For profit	121947	43628 (36)	19473 (30)
>100 beds	131631	46393 (35)	16708 (30)
Part of a chain	102224	35870 (35)	27231 (32)
>80% Medicaid beds	30731	13372 (44)	49729 (32)
Residents with a do-not-resuscitate order, %			
<10	13847	6749 (49)	56352 (33)
11–20	19198	9204 (48)	53897 (32)
21–40	46892	19191 (41)	43910 (31)
41–60	48640	15707 (32)	47394 (34)

Table 10.2. Multivariate Analysis of Resident and Facility Characteristics Associated With Tube-Fed Residents With Advanced Cognitive Impairment in US Nursing Homes

Characteristic	OR (95% CI)
Resident Characteristics (N = 186 835)	
Age, y	
<65	1.77 (1.71–1.83)
65–69	1.32 (1.27–1.38)
70–74	1.26 (1.22–1.30)
75–79	1.24 (1.21–1.27)
80–84	1.17 (1.15–1.21)
85–90	1.15 (1.12–1.18)
≥90	1.00
Men	1.15 (1.14–1.18)
Race or ethnicity	
White (not of Hispanic origin)	1.00
American Indian/Alaska Native	1.17 (1.04–1.30)
Hispanic	1.30 (1.24–1.36)

continued

Table 10.2. *(continued)*

Characteristic	OR (95% CI)*
Black (not of Hispanic origin)	1.55 (1.51–1.58)
Asian/Pacific Islander	1.57 (1.46–1.67)
Marital status	
Married	1.00
Never married	1.01 (0.99–1.04)
Widowed	0.96 (0.95–0.98)
Separated	0.99 (0.93–1.05)
Divorced	1.06 (1.03–1.10)
Absent	
Do-not-resuscitate order	1.07 (1.06–1.10)
Durable power of attorney for health care	1.19 (1.16–1.22)
Living will	1.32 (1.28–1.35)
Diagnosis of Alzheimer disease	1.37 (1.34–1.40)
Diagnosis of cancer	1.08 (1.04–1.11)
Present	
Diagnosis of stroke	1.84 (1.82–1.86)
Recent decline in functional status	1.04 (1.01–1.06)
Facility Characteristics (N = 15135)	
No dementia special care unit	1.11 (1.07–1.15)
Urban location	1.14 (1.11–1.16)
For profit	1.09 (1.06–1.12)
>100 beds	1.04 (1.01–1.07)
Part of a chain	0.96 (0.94–1.00)
>80% Medicaid beds	1.00 (0.97–1.03)
Residents with a do-not-resuscitate order, %	
<10	1.67 (1.54–1.80)
11–20	1.69 (1.56–1.81)
21–40	1.54 (1.44–1.65)
41–60	1.37 (1.28–1.47)
61–80	1.22 (1.13–1.30)
>80	1.00
Nonwhite residents, %	
0	1.00

Resident Characteristics

Our multivariate analysis identified several resident characteristics that were independently associated with feeding tube use in advanced cognitive impairment. Residents who were younger and male were more likely to have feeding tubes. The likelihood of feeding tube use was lowest among white residents. Marital status was also independently associated with feeding tube use. Divorced residents with advanced cognitive impairment had a greater likelihood of feeding tube use compared with married residents.

A greater proportion of severely cognitively impaired residents with feeding tubes did not have advance directives compared with residents without feeding tubes. The lack of a DNR order, no durable power of attorney for health care, and no living will were independently associated with feeding-tube status in the multivariate model.

Residents without a diagnosis of Alzheimer disease were more likely to have feeding tubes compared with other residents with advanced cognitive impairment. A history of stroke was associated with a greater likelihood of having a feeding tube, while residents with cancer were less likely to have a feeding tube. Finally, a recent decline in functional status was independently associated with feeding tube use.

Facility Characteristics

Several demographic, organizational, and fiscal features of nursing homes were independently associated with feeding tube use (Table 2). Residents in facilities lacking a dementia special care unit had a greater likelihood of feeding tube use compared with residents in facilities with these units. In addition, individuals were more likely to have feeding tubes if they lived in nursing homes that were in located in an urban setting, were run for profit, and that had more than 100 beds. Chain ownership was not associated with feeding-tube status.

Residents in facilities with more than 80% of their beds dedicated to Medicaid recipients were more likely to receive feeding tubes compared with patients who resided in nursing homes with fewer beds dedicated to Medicaid recipients. However, this relationship was not sustained after controlling for other residents and facility characteristics. This association was confounded primarily by the racial or ethnic profile of the facility, such that nursing homes with a greater proportion of nonwhites were more likely to have more than 80% of beds dedicated to Medicaid recipients and also to have residents with feeding tubes.

Advance directives were independently associated with feeding-tube status at the facility level. Older persons with advanced cognitive impairment residing in nursing homes in which a relatively smaller proportion of the resident population had DNR orders had a greater likelihood of having a feeding tube. For example, feeding tube use was more likely in facilities in which the prevalence of DNR orders was 61%-80% compared with facilities in which more than 80% of residents had DNR orders (OR, 1.22, 95%; CI, 1.13–1.30). This significant trend persisted in a dose-response fashion as the frequency of DNR orders decreased.

The racial or ethnic profile of the facility was also independently associated with the use of feeding tubes. Compared with nursing homes with white residents only, feeding tube use was more likely to occur in facilities with higher proportions of nonwhite residents.

The lack of a nurse practitioner or physician assistant on the nursing home staff was independently associated with a higher likelihood of feeding tube use among residents with advanced cognitive impairment (OR, 1.07; 95% Cl, 1.04–1.10). Other staffing variables, including the ratio of licensed nurses and nursing assistants per bed and having a speech therapist on staff, were not associated with the use of feeding tubes after multivariate adjustment.

Residents were more likely to receive feeding tubes if they lived in facilities that had higher rates of new admissions with feeding tubes. The facility rate of residents receiving intravenous therapy was not associated with feeding-tube status.

Feeding Tube Use within Nursing Homes in Each State

Figure 1 presents the facility rates of feeding tube use among nursing home residents with advanced cognitive impairment in each state. Figure 1 highlights the variation in practice across facilities both within and among states. For example, in Tennessee, the use of feeding tubes among residents with advanced cognitive impairment is less than 16% in 24% of facilities; ranges from 16%–40% in 42% of facilities exceeds 40% in 34% of facilities. The District of Columbia had the highest proportion (90%) of nursing homes in which the use of feeding tubes exceeded 40%.

The number of nursing homes in each state and the proportion of tube-fed residents with severe cognitive impairment in each state are presented in the columns beside the Figure 1. The prevalence of feeding tube use at the individual level was also the highest in the District of Columbia where 64% of residents have feeding tubes.

COMMENT

This nationwide study demonstrates that the use of feeding tubes among nursing home residents with severe cognitive impairment is common and associated not only with their clinical features, but with the fiscal, organizational, demographic, and ethnic or racial profile of the facility in which they live. The relative influence of these nursing home characteristics is further demonstrated by the observation that feeding tube practice varies considerably among facilities within the same state. We identified several potentially modifiable factors at the facility level that may reduce feeding tube use, including

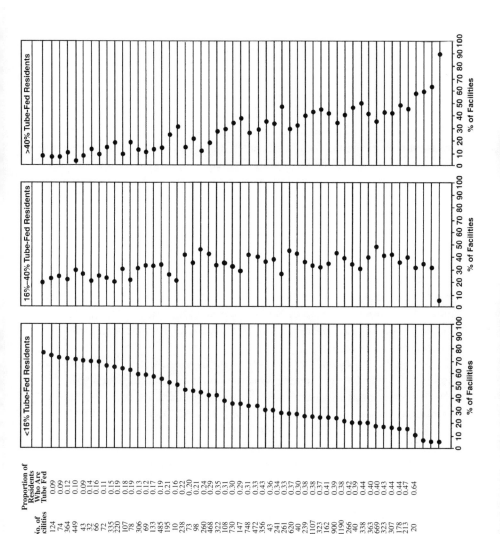

State	No. of Facilities	Proportion of Residents Who Are Tube Fed
Me	124	0.09
NH	74	0.09
Minn	364	0.12
Iowa	449	0.10
Vt	43	0.09
Wyo	32	0.14
Mont	66	0.16
ND	72	0.11
Kan	335	0.15
Neb	220	0.19
SD	107	0.18
Utah	78	0.19
Wis	306	0.13
Idaho	69	0.12
Ore	133	0.17
Mass	485	0.19
Colo	195	0.21
Alaska	10	0.16
Conn	238	0.22
NM	73	0.20
RI	98	0.21
Wash	260	0.24
Mo	468	0.29
Mich	322	0.35
WVa	108	0.31
Ill	730	0.30
Ariz	147	0.29
Pa	748	0.31
Ind	472	0.33
Okla	356	0.43
Hawaii	43	0.36
Ark	241	0.34
Va	261	0.33
NY	620	0.37
Del	40	0.30
Md	239	0.38
Tex	1107	0.38
Tenn	323	0.37
SC	162	0.41
Ohio	900	0.39
Calif	1190	0.38
Ky	266	0.42
Nev	40	0.39
NJ	338	0.44
NC	363	0.40
Fla	669	0.40
Ga	323	0.43
La	307	0.44
Miss	178	0.44
Ala	213	0.47
DC	20	0.64

greater use of advance directives, having a nurse practitioner or physician assistant on staff, and having a special dementia care unit.

This study supports and extends earlier work examining factors associated with feeding tube use in the institutionalized elderly with advanced cognitive impairment.[4–5, 7–9] However, this investigation is unique in several important ways. First, the study includes residents from all licensed US nursing homes. Second, it is the only study to examine both resident and facility characteristics in a single analytic model. Only one other investigation has comprehensively examined nursing homes' characteristics associated with the use of feeding tubes in this population. However, this earlier study is limited because it only examined facility characteristics associated with the overall rate of feeding tube use at the facility level; it did not consider resident characteristics in the model; data from only 6 states were included; and several important facility factors were not analyzed. Finally, our use of the generalized estimating equation approach to adjust for correlations among residents in the same nursing home make the findings even more robust.

Using a national data set, our findings corroborate many previously reported correlates of patient characteristics associated with feeding tube use among individuals with advanced cognitive impairments including younger age[5, 8–9], no diagnosis of Alzheimer disease[5, 8–9], stroke[5, 8–9], lack of advance directives to limit aggressive care,[5, 8–9] and nonwhite race[5, 7, 9]. Some studies, including ours, found an increase in feeding tube use among men, while others reported the opposite.[5]

Among the most notable observations in this study is the increased likelihood of feeding tube use among residents living in for-profit nursing homes. This observation is consistent with the notion put forward in the lay and scientific press that feeding tube use among patients with advanced cognitive impairment may be used by nursing homes as a means of cost-saving.[16–19] The staff's time required for feeding residents by hand is expensive.[18–19] In addition, Medicaid reimbursement schemes in many states pay higher per diem rates for tube-fed residents compared with similarly debilitated residents who do not have feeding tubes.[18, 20] However, Medicaid payments have been shown not to be associated with feeding tube use at the state level.[3] Moreover, the practice varies greatly among nursing homes even within the same state. Therefore, while the potential for financial incentives to favor use of feeding tubes exists, this association remains to be proven.

Previous work has shown that the use of DNR orders is strongly associated with feeding tube use in patients with advanced cognitive impairment at both the patient[5, 8–9] and state levels.[3] This study underscores the important role of DNR orders at the nursing home level.[4] The association between higher facility rates of DNR orders with a lower likelihood of feeding tube use deserves further investigation. One potential explanation is that facilities with a greater overall rate of DNR orders may be more proficient at engaging surrogates in discussions that lead to decisions not to use a feeding tube. In addition, families that request DNR orders may also be less likely to want to have a feeding tube used. The MDS is unable to provide any information about the decision-making process between families and health care providers.

This study demonstrates that the role of race or ethnicity in end-of-life decision making extends beyond the background of the individual patient. It has been widely reported that nonwhites tend to choose more aggressive end-of-life care,[21-22] including the use of feeding tubes.[5,7,9] Possible explanations for this observation include different cultural attitudes toward death and dying, apprehension of nonwhites toward the medical system, and poor communication of advance directives to minorities by health care providers. The racial or ethnic mix of the nursing home may be linked to other facility factors that influence feeding tube use that we were unable to measure, such as the background of the nursing home staff. Black physicians are less likely to view feeding tube use in advanced dementia as a heroic measure.[23]

This study confirms that severely cognitively impaired residents living in nursing homes that are larger[4], located in urban areas[9], and lack dementia special care units[4] have a greater likelihood of using feeding tubes. The closer proximity of urban nursing homes to tertiary medical centers may translate into an increased use of high technology care at the end of life.[24] On the other hand, fewer feeding tubes among nursing home residents with access to dementia special care units suggests that these units may have greater success at guiding care toward palliation. We also found that facilities that had either a nurse practitioner or physician assistant on staff were less likely to have patients using feeding tubes. Some data suggest that clinicians who practice solely in nursing homes may be less likely to promote feeding tube use among residents with advanced dementia compared with community-based clinicians.[25]

This study has several limitations that deserve comment. Some resident and facility characteristics that may be associated with feeding tube use were not available in the MDS and OSCAR data sets, such as religious affiliation, characteristics of the nursing home staff, and facility-specific policies regarding artificial nutrition and hydration. We also lacked information about the quality of counseling between practitioners and families regarding the use of feeding tubes in individuals with advanced cognitive impairment. In addition, the MDS and OSCAR data may include some inaccuracies. However, any inaccuracies would be likely to bias results toward the null. Finally, while we were able to identify the pattern of feeding tube use in the United States in 1999, it is possible that policies have since been introduced that have changed the observed behavior.

The aggressiveness of care provided at the end of life is increasingly recognized to be determined by more than the preferences and needs of individual patients.[24, 26] This study confirms that feeding tube use among older persons with advanced cognitive impairment varies depending on the characteristics of the nursing home in which they reside. As such, our findings highlight potential interventions and policy changes at the facility level that could influence this practice. Comprehensive implementation of advanced care planning is likely to reduce the use of feeding tubes. However, future research will need to explore how the facilities' rates of DNR orders relate to the broader process of shared decision making. Moreover, if financial incentives are proven to favor feeding tube use, then reimbursement policies that promote feeding by hand should be considered. Feeding tube use may also be reduced by having providers and units dedicated to the care of nursing home residents with advanced cognitive impairment. Finally, a greater understanding of the influence of race or ethnicity on the use of feeding tubes is needed to ensure informed and culturally sensitive decisions for all residents.

AUTHOR INFORMATION

Corresponding Author and Reprints: Susan L. Mitchell, MD, MPH, Hebrew Rehabilitation Center for Aged, 1200 Centre St, Boston, MA 02131 (e-mail: smitchell@mail.hrca.harvard.edu).
Author Contributions. *Study concept and design:* Mitchell, Teno, Kabumoto, Mor.
Acquisition of data: Mitchell, Teno, Mor.
Analysis and interpretation of data: Mitchell, Teno, Roy, Kabumoto, Mor.
Drafting of the manuscript: Mitchell, Teno, Roy, Kabumoto, Mor.
Critical revision of the manuscript for important intellectual content: Mitchell, Teno, Roy, Mor.
Statistical expertise: Mitchell, Teno, Roy, Kabumoto, Mor.
Obtained funding: Teno, Mor.
Administrative, technical, or material support: Mitchell, Teno, Roy, Kabumoto, Mor.
Study supervision: Mitchell, Teno, Mor.

Funding/Support: Dr Mitchell is supported by the National Institutes of Health and National Institute on Aging Mentored Patient Research Award (K23AG20054–01) and the Marcus Applebaum Fund at Hebrew Rehabilitation Center for Aged. Dr Mor is supported by a National Institute on Aging

MERIT Award (11624). This work was supported by grant 037188 from the Robert Wood Johnson Foundation.
Author Affiliations: Hebrew Rehabilitation Center for Aged Research and Training Institute, Department of Medicine, Beth Israel Deaconess Medical Center, and Division on Aging, Harvard Medical School, Boston, Mass (Dr. Mitchell); and Center for Gerontology and Health Care Research, Department of Community Health, Brown Medical School, Providence, RI (Drs. Teno, Roy, and Mor and Mr Kabumoto).

NOTES

1. Finucane TE, Christmas C, Travis K. Tube feeding in patients with advanced dementia: a review of the evidence. *JAMA.* 1999;282:1365–1370. ABSTRACT/ FULL TEXT

2. Gillick MR. Rethinking the role of tube feeding in patients with advanced dementia. *N Engl J Med.* 2000; 342:206–210. FULL TEXT

3. Teno JM, Mor V, DeSilva D, Kabumoto G, Roy J, Wetle T. Use of feeding tubes in nursing home residents with severe cognitive impairment. *JAMA.* 2002;287:3211–3212. FULL TEXT

4. Mitchell SL, Kiely DK, Gillick MR. Nursing home characteristics associated with tube feeding in advanced cognitive impairment. *J Am Geriatr Soc.* 2003; 51:75–79. MEDLINE

5. Ahronheim JC, Mulvihill M, Sieger C, et al. State practice variations in the use of tube feeding for nursing home residents with severe cognitive impairment. *J Am Geriatr Soc.* 2001;49:148–152. MEDLINE

6. Mitchell MD SL, Kiely MPH DK. A cross-national comparison of institutionalized tube-fed older persons. *J Am Med Dir Assoc.* 2001; 2:10–14. MEDLINE

7. Meier DE, Ahronheim JC, Morris J, et al. High short-term mortality in hospitalized patients with advanced dementia. *Arch Intern Med.* 2001;161:594–599. ABSTRACT/FULL TEXT

8. Mitchell SL, Kiely DK, Lipsitz LA. The risk factors and impact on survival of feeding tubes in nursing home residents with severely advanced dementia. *Arch Intern Med.* 1997; 157:327–332. ABSTRACT

9. Gessert CE, Mosier MC, Brown EF, Frey B. Tube feeding in nursing home residents with severe and irreversible cognitive impairment. *J Am Geriatr Soc.* 2000;48:1593–1600. ISI / MEDLINE

10. Intrator O, Castle NG, Mor V. Facility characteristics associated with hospitalization of nursing home residents. *Med Care.* 1999;37:228–237. CrossRef ISI / MEDLINE

11. Morris JN, Hawes C, Fries BE, et al. Designing the national assessment instrument for nursing homes. *Gerontologist.* 1990;30:293–307. ABSTRACT

12. Morris JN, Fries BE, Mehr DR, et al. MDS Cognitive Performance Scale. *J Gerontol.* 1994;49:M174– M182. ISI / MEDLINE

13. Hartmaier SL, Sloane PD, Guess HA, et al. Validation of the Minimum Data Set Cognitive Performance Scale. *J Gerontol A Biol Sci Med Sci.* 1995;50:MI28–MI33. ISI / MEDLINE

14. SAS Institute Inc. *SAS/STAT Software: Changes and Enhancement Through Release 6.12.* Cary, NC: SAS Institute Inc; 1997.

15. Zhang J, Yu KF. What's the relative risk? a method of correcting the odds ratio in cohort studies of common outcomes. *JAMA.* 1998;280:1690–1691. ABSTRACT/ FULL TEXT

16. Mitchell SL. Financial incentives to place feeding tubes in nursing home residents with advanced dementia. *J Am Geriatr Soc.* 2003; 51:129–131. ISI / MEDLINE

17. Grady D. Calls growing for stopping tube feeding in dementia. *New York Times.* January 20, 2000:A13.

18. Mitchell MD SL, Buchanan JL, Littlehale S, Hamel M. Tube-feeding versus hand-feeding nursing home residents with advanced dementia: a cost comparison. *J Am Med Dir Assoc.* 2003;4:27–33. MEDLINE

19. Kayser-Jones J, Schell ES, Porter C, et al. Factors contributing to dehydration in nursing homes. *Geriatr Soc.* 1999;47:1187–1194. ISI / MEDLINE

20. Fries BE, Schneider DP, Foley WJ, et al. Refining a case-mix index measure for nursing homes. *Med Care.* 1994;32:668–685. ISI / MEDLINE

21. Blackhall LJ, Frank G, Murphy ST, Michel V, Palmer J, Azen SP. Ethnicity and attitudes towards life sustaining technology. *Soc Sci Med.* 1999;48:1779–1789. Cross-Ref / ISI / MEDLINE

22. Kiely DK, Mitchell SL, Marlow A, et al. Ethnic differences in advance directives in nursing home residents. *J Am Geriatr Soc.* 2001;49:1346–1352. ISI / MEDLINE

23. Mebane EW, Oman RF, Kroonen LT, Goldstein MK. The influence of physician race, age and gender on physician attitudes towards advance directives and preferences for end-of-life decision-making. *Geriatr Soc.* 1999;47:579–591. ISI / MEDLINE

24. Pritchard RS, Fisher ES, Teno JM, et al. Influence of patient preferences and local health systems characteristics on the place of death. *J Am Geriatr Soc.* 1998;46:1242–1250. ISI /MEDLINE

25. Batchelor AL, Winsemius D, O'Connor PJ, Wetle T. Predictors of advance directive restrictiveness and compliance with institutional policies in long-term care facilities. *J Am Geriatr Soc.* 1992;40:679. MEDLINE

26. Meier DE, Morrison RS. Autonomy reconsidered. *N Engl J Med.* 2002; 346:1087–1088. FULL TEXT

11

Xenografts and Retroviruses

Robin A. Weiss

"Uncertain peril and certain promise" was how Joshua Lederberg described the new recombinant DNA technology when molecular biologists met in 1975 to impose a short-lived moratorium on genetic engineering. The same epithet applies today to xenotransplantation, the grafting of animal cells and tissues into humans.[1] Xenotransplantation, too, has led to calls for a moratorium[2] so that the ethical issues involved[3] and the hazards of cross-species infection can be publicly debated. Some reassurance on safety is provided on page 1236 of this issue[4] by a consortium of investigators from Novartis and the Centers for Disease Control and Prevention (CDC). Paradis *et al.* report that infection by porcine endogenous retrovirus (PERV)—one potential risk of transplanting patients with pig tissues—does not appear to have occurred in any of 160 persons exposed to living pig cells.[4]

The "certain promise" is that xenotransplantation could provide a ready supply of cells, tissues, and organs to treat a variety of serious human conditions. The "uncertain perils" are to what extent the animal cells or tissue will perform properly in the human host, whether immunological rejection can be overcome, and whether harmful zoonoses (animal-to-human infections) can be prevented.[1, 3] Despite the greater immunological barrier, pigs are favored over primates as a source of transplant tissue for a variety of practical, ethical, and safety reasons. Among the many microbes harbored by pigs, PERV has aroused particular concern. Animal endogenous retroviruses are integrated proviral DNA genomes inherited in a Mendelian manner. At least 50 copies of PERV exist in pig chromosomes and PERV cannot be eliminated by pathogen-free, closed breeding of pigs. Some PERV genomes have given rise to human-tropic PERV strains in culture.[5, 6]

Fetal pig nerve cells have been transplanted into patients' brains in an attempt to slow down neurodegeneration in Parkinson's and Huntington's diseases[7] and to treat epilepsy. A recent report on 24 such patients indicated no evidence of subsequent PERV infection in the blood.[8] Last year, lack of PERV infection was reported in 10 diabetic patients transplanted with pig pancreatic islet cells secreting insulin[9] and in two renal dialysis patients whose blood was extracorporeally perfused through pig kidneys.[10] Eight of the diabetics and both of the dialysis patients were reanalyzed in the present 160–patient study,[4] which used similar PCR and RT-PCR amplification methods to detect viral genomes, and Western blotting to detect viral antigens in serum (see the table).

The lack of evidence for PERV infection will encourage biotechnology companies, physicians, and surgeons to explore pig tissue treatments further. For example (as reported for one patient by Paradis *et al.*), circulation of human blood across porcine hepatocytes in culture is under investigation as a treatment for patients with acute liver failure.[4] Of course, a major goal is to make up for the shortage of available human organs for transplantation by supplying pig kidneys and hearts instead. But hyperacute rejection and acute vascular rejection present a major hurdle to whole-organ xenotransplantation.[1, 3] Rejection of pig organs is triggered by natural human antibodies that recognize carbohydrate "xeno-antigens"—mainly α^{1-3} galactose-expressed on pig endothelial cells that line blood vessels.[11] Several biotechnology companies are attempting to block complement-mediated immune attack of xenografts by breeding transgenic pigs that express human proteins.[1] But an unfortunate corollary of such genetically modified pigs may be that the porcine viruses they carry may more readily infect humans.[12]

The most striking scientific finding reported by Paradis *et al.* is the apparent long-term survival of porcine cells in the blood of 23 of 100 patients in St. Petersburg, Russia, whose blood had been perfused through pig spleens for 1 hour up to 8 years previously. Survival of transplanted donor cells in the recipient is known as microchimerism, and it can confound the sensitive detection of PERV infection. In fact, the Novartis/CDC study only examined microchimerism in those patients who first yielded a PERV-positive result; in other words, the 50 copies of retroviral DNA naturally resident in the pig genome were used as first-line detection of pig cell microchimerism. Extremely low numbers of pig cells (<1 per 100,000 human cells) were estimated to be present in the human samples. However, only 4 of the 23 samples tested by both Novartis and CDC were PERV-positive, which raises the question of PCR contamination (the bane of all highly sensitive forensic or diagnostic DNA amplification tests). The long-term survival of pig cells detected as pig DNA in the patients' circulation is surprising in view of a report on pig-to-baboon microchimerism indicating that the pig cells become rapidly sequestered from the circulating blood.[13]

Paradis *et al.* do not state the ailments for which the Russian patients were subjected to "immunotherapy" by spleen extracorporeal perfusion. One wonders whether the physicians conducting this procedure ever stop to consider a risk-benefit analysis of passing their patients' blood through the spleens of farm pigs fresh from the abattoir and whether they inform the patients of the risk of infection. Nevertheless, the Russian data provide us with evidence for a lack of PERV infection despite apparent long-term survival of pig viruses in the human body. It will surely be most important to test these patients for evidence of infection by other prevalent systemic pig viruses such as porcine parvovirus and porcine circovirus, which are unlikely to be wholly excluded from closed breeding herds.

A chain of events required for PERV to pose a threat to public health has been proposed.[14] PERV is present in the pigs being bred for xenotransplantation, and human-tropic PERV is expressed in many cells and tissues,[5, 6] though apparently not in fetal brain cells.[8] Thus far, PERV has not infected patients exposed to porcine tissues,[4, 8–10] but if this were to occur, we would need to investigate whether PERV caused disease and whether it could be transmitted to other individuals. To address the risks of infection, the U.S. Food and Drug Administration (FDA) established an Advisory Panel on Xenotransplantation. And in 1997, the British government, still reeling from the evidence that bovine spongiform encephalopathy ("mad cow disease") had spread to humans, moved quickly to set up the UK Xenotransplantation Interim Regulatory Authority (UKXIRA).

With the latest reports[4, 8] on the lack of evidence for PERV infection in vivo, the keenest advocates of xenotransplantation may mutter that the concern over the risk of PERV infection unnecessarily delayed progress in the field. The Novartis/CDC teams, however, conclude that only cautious progress in closely monitored, prospective clinical trials will help in "assessing the safety and efficacy of using porcine cells, tissues, or organs therapeutically in humans."[4] Both the FDA and UKXIRA take this attitude and appear ready to approve, in principle, small-scale human trials of porcine cellular therapy.

Whereas the endogenous retroviruses in our house guests (cats and mice) have not naturally been transmitted to humans, we have known for more than 20 years that human tumor xenografts grown in immunosuppressed animals sometimes become infected.[15] PERV, however, does not proliferate as readily in human cells as human-tropic feline and murine endogenous retroviruses.[5, 6] But the possibility remains that, say, one among 1000 xenograft recipients may become infected by PERV or by a virus resulting from recombination between PERV and human retroviral sequences.

The concern, then, will be the potential for onward transmission from the rare, infected transplant recipient to his or her contacts. Lest we dismiss this notion as ridiculous, we should bear in mind that HIV-1 began as a zoonosis, probably from chimpanzees, and that the worldwide pandemic of the major

HIV-1 subgroups may be attributable to a single cross-species event.[16] Neither can we be sure that AIDS did not have an iatrogenic (medically caused) origin, if chimpanzee kidneys were used in Africa to propagate certain batches of poliovirus vaccine.[17]

Although the public may demand evidence of no risk, retrospective epidemiological surveys can at best provide no evidence of risk, which is a rather different matter. We should heed the Hippocratic precautionary principle—"at least do no harm." Yet no new medical procedure can be deemed entirely safe, so we need to balance risk with benefit, for the patient and for the human population.

For the individual transplant recipient, the real promise seems to be greater than uncertain peril. Indeed, one of the potential advantages of xenotransplantation over allotransplantation (person-to-person grafts) is that pathogen-free pigs might pose a lesser threat of infection than a graft from an unknown human donor. After all, many cases of life-threatening infections have been transmitted by human transplantation and transfusion: HIV, hepatitis B and C viruses, various herpesviruses, tuberculosis, and Creutzfeldt-Jakob disease.

For the community at large, the risk-benefit equation is much more difficult to quantify. It took more than 20 years for HIV-1 to spread out of Africa, and it is only after 55 years of individual benefit from antibiotics that we are facing the public health threat of multidrug-resistant microbes. The ethical and technical problems of maintaining vigilance over xenotransplantation should not be underestimated.

Table. 11.1.   Detection of Perv in Human Tissue and Serum

Reverse transcriptase (RT) activity[4,9]

> Product-enhanced (amplified) RT assays detect < 100 particles ml⁻¹ but are not PERV-specific.

Viral genome sequences[4, 8–10]

> PERV-specific amplification of proviral DNA in cells by polymerase chain reaction (PCR) detects < 10 PERV genomes with high specificity.

> RT-PCR, DNA synthesis, and amplification from [4, 9] viral RNA in plasma detects < 50 PERV genomes ml⁻¹ with high specificity.

Antiviral antibodies

> Western blot detects recombinant Gag viral[4, 9] antigen, whole virus, or infected cell lysate.

> Enzyme-linked immunosorbent assay (ELISA) detects Gag antigen or whole virus. Expected to be more sensitive though slightly less specific than Western blot.

> Neutralization of virus distinguishes between [10] envelope variants of infectious PERV[6] but probably less sensitive than ELISA or Western blot.

NOTES

1. H. Auchinloss and D. H. Sachs, *Annu. Rev. Immunol.* 16, 433 (1998); R. A. Weiss, *Br. Med, J.* 317, 931 (1998).

2. F. H. Bach et al., *Nature Med.* 4, 141 (1998); D. Butler, *Nature* 391, 320 (1998).

3. *Animal-to-Human Transplants: The Ethics of Xenotransplantation* (Nuffield Council on Bioethics, London, 1996); *Xenotransplantation, Science, Ethics and Public Policy* (Institute of Medicine, Washington, DC, 1996); Department of Health Advisory Group on the Ethics of Xenotransplantation, *Animal Tissues into Humans* (Her Majesty's Stationary Office, London, 1997); J. Fishman, D. Sachs, R. Shaikh, Eds., *Xenotransplantation: Scientific Frontiers and Public Policy, Ann. N.Y. Acad. Sci.* 862, 1 (1998).

4. K. Paradis *et al., Science* 285, 1236 (1999).

5. C. Patience, Y. Takeuchi, R. A. Weiss, *Nature Med.* 3, 282 (1997); C. Wilson *et al., J. Virol* 72, 3082 (1998); U. Martin *et al., Lancet* 352, 692 (1998).

6. P. Le Tissier *et al., Nature* 389, 681 (1997); Y. Takeuchi *et al., J. Virol.* 72, 9986 (1998).

7. T. Deacon *et al., Nature Med* 3, 350 (1997); S. A. Ellias et al., *Mov. Disord.* 12, 839 (1997); M. St. Hiltaire *et al., Neurology* 50, S10.008 (1998).

8. J. H. Dinsmore *et al.,* Presented at the Food and Drug Administration Advisory Panel on Xenotransplantation, Washington, DC, June 1999.

9. W. Heneine *et al., Lancet* 352, 695 (1998).

10. C. Patience et al., *ibid.,* p. 699.

11. R. P. Rother and S. P. Squinto, *Cell* 86, 185 (1996).

12. R. A. Weiss, *Nature* 391, 327 (1998).

13. C. W. Hoopes and J. L. Platt, *Transplantation* 64, 347 (1997).

14. J. P. Stoye, *Lancet* 352, 666 (1998).

15. B. G. Achong, B. G. Trumper, B. C. Giovanella, *Br. J. Cancer* 34, 203 (1976); R. A. Weiss, *Natl. Cancer. Inst. Monogr.* 48, 183 (1978).

16. F. Gao *et al., Nature* 397, 436 (1999); R. A. Weiss and R. W. Wrangham, *ibid.,* p. 385; T. Zhu et al., *ibid.* 391, 594 (1998).

17. E. Hooper, *The River. A Journey to the Source of HIV and AIDS* (Little, Brown & Co., New York, 1999).

12

Donating Spare Embryos for Embryonic Stem-Cell Research

Ethics Committee of the American Society for Reproductive Medicine

The ability to isolate and culture human embryonic stem (ES) cells, which was first reported in 1998, has opened a promising area of medical research.[1] Derived from the inner cell mass of blastocyst-stage embryos, pluripotent ES cells give rise to all cell types in the human body and are thought to be able to proliferate indefinitely in an undifferentiated state.[2] Researchers predict that, if coaxed to differentiate in culture, ES cells can be used to create specialized cells to treat a wide range of diseases and conditions, including Parkinson's disease, Alzheimer's disease, cancer, spinal cord injury, and juvenile-onset diabetes. Other envisioned uses of ES cells include research to understand cell specialization and the development and testing of new drugs.[3]

Human ES cell research has provoked considerable discussion about ethics and policy. Among other commissions, the National Bioethics Advisory Commission considered the question of federal funding of ES cell research in 1999 and recommended that the government fund both the derivation and use of ES cells from spare, donated embryos. The Clinton administration proposed funding only the use of ES cells, and the National Institutes of Health subsequently issued guidelines to oversee the process. Before any grants were made, however, a change of administration occurred. After further review of the issue, President Bush announced on August 9, 2001, that the administration would consider for funding only those proposals using human ES cells from cell lines that had been derived and cultured by August 9, 2001.[4]

Although this decision opened the door to fundable research, many scientists have questioned whether the preexisting cell lines would be adequate for the research or therapies to which they might lead. Privately funded investigators are likely to seek additional donated embryos in order to obtain new ES cell lines for research in their own laboratories. New sources of embryos will enable investigators to study the derivation process itself, secure more cells from the initial embryo source if necessary, and culture cell lines from varied genetic sources. In addition, the human ES cells derived before August 9, 2001, were cultured in their undifferentiated state on a feeder layer of embryonic mouse cells, which will render these cell lines unacceptable for clinical trials. Presumably, new cell lines will be needed for clinical trials to commence.

A primary source of embryos for future ES cell research is likely to be embryos donated by couples undergoing IVF who no longer want or need their embryos for fertility treatment. We consider here the conditions under which fertility clinics and other facilities that store embryos may ethically make embryos available for researchers seeking ES cells. This consideration is preceded by a summary of differing perspectives about the ethics of embryo research.

ETHICS OF HUMAN EMBRYO RESEARCH

Human embryo research has elicited diverse and conflicting perspectives since the early days of in vitro fertilization. Discussions about the human embryo are frequently framed in terms of the embryo's moral status. An important distinction arises between those who regard the embryo as a person, with all the protections accorded fellow members of the human community, and those who regard the embryo as deserving respect as a potential human being but not the same respect accorded persons.

Those who believe the embryo has the moral status of persons expect that the embryo should be accorded all the rights of these individuals. Under this perspective, the embryo is vulnerable and needs protection. Some believe this status begins during fertilization, when the DNA from the female and male gametes combines to create an entity with a novel genetic composition. Others believe the status begins later, when the primitive streak begins to develop approximately 14 days after fertilization and when the embryo will, if it survives, develop into a single individual.

Most of those who believe that the embryo has a lesser status than adults and children regard the embryo as a potential human being worthy of special respect but not entitled to the same rights as persons. According to this perspective, the embryo used in research ranges in size from a single cell to hundreds of cells with no nervous system and a limited chance of developing to birth. The possibility of twinning or regression to a nonviable entity up to the 14th day after fertilization is consistent with the notion that the embryo lacks individuality. Moreover. according to this point of view, the early embryo lacks the criteria traditionally equated with human status.

The Ethics Committee of the American Society for Reproductive Medicine (ASRM) has consistently held to the second perspective, which regards the embryo as a potential human being worthy of special respect.[5-8] The ASRM Ethics Committee regards embryo research as ethically acceptable if it is likely to provide significant new knowledge that will benefit human health and if it is conducted in ways that accord the embryo respect. The Ethics Committee, along with commissions and advisory bodies from around the world, has developed core expectations about how research using embryos may ethically be conducted.[8, 9] Among other things, couples must give informed consent to donate their spare embryos for research, embryos should not be kept cleaving more than 14 days after fertilization, and there should be no buying and selling of embryos. It is also expected that the investigator bears the burden of justifying the worthiness of the research, uses the smallest possible number of embryos, submits proposals to review by an institutional review board, has no satisfactory alternative to using embryos, and expects important clinical data to accrue from the research.

The ability of scientists to isolate and culture human ES cells has evoked renewed discussions about the ethics of embryo research. Advocates of ES cell research argue that preimplantation embryos will be discarded in any event and it is appropriate to gain some benefit from the act. In light of the potentially significant impact on regenerative medicine, they argue it may even be morally obligatory to pursue this research. They also note that donation for embryo research is an extension of the couple's authority over the disposition of embryos.

Critics, on the other hand, argue that research causing the destruction of embryos is wrong. In addition, they argue that adult stem cells also hold potential for diagnostics and therapy. They also express concern that the research will lead to the treatment of embryos as commodities and, consequently to diminished respect for embryos. The matter of whether embryos may ethically be created for ES cell research through in vitro fertilization or somatic cell nuclear transfer remains a topic of continued debate and elusive consensus.[10-15]

INFORMED CONSENT AND THE DONATION OF SPARE EMBRYOS FOR ES CELL RESEARCH

A distinct feature of ES cell investigations is the intent to derive cell lines that may continue to divide indefinitely and be used by researchers for many years to come. Cell lines eventually may have considerable commercial value. In addition they may potentially be traced to donors.[10] For these and other reasons, it is appropriate to revisit guidelines about what should be conveyed to couples in the donation process, when, and by whom. These guidelines aim to protect the autonomous interests of couples faced with deciding the disposition of embryos they no longer want or need.

What Information to Convey to Potential Donors

Informed consent is a basic requirement for the ethical conduct of all human subjects research, including, studies using human embryos. Couples who donate embryos for research should be told of the risks and benefits of donation. For example, a risk might arise if the couple were later to wish they still had the embryos available for their fertility efforts. A benefit might be the satisfaction of knowing they have contributed to research designed to advance medical therapies. Couples should also be told of the purpose and nature of the research and of whether the research is expected to have commercial value. They should be told that they may change their mind about donation at any time until the experiment begins, that their status in the infertility program will not be affected if they do not donate spare embryos, and that no embryos used in the study will be transferred for pregnancy.[8]

In the case of donation for ES cell research, other considerations may also be relevant. Given the wide range of uses to which ES cells may be put, couples should be informed of the specific research project, if known, or at least of the category of anticipated research, such as reproductive research, development of therapies for disease, or product development. Couples should also know that ES cell research typically involves deriving cells from the inner cell mass of an embryo at the blastocyst stage, which leads to the embryo's destruction.

Potential donors also should be informed that cell lines might exist indefinitely. They should be told that stem cells from embryos may have commercial value for a wide range of research and clinical purpose, and that they as donors will not share in the commercial value. The clinic should develop a policy on privacy and confidentiality of donations and present this as part of the consent process. If identifiers are attached to the cell lines, the donors must be informed of this and of steps taken to assure their anonymity. The male and female partners must agree on the disposition of their spare embryos. If they cannot jointly agree to donate embryos for research, the embryos should not be used for research.

When Consent Should Be Obtained

It is important that couples decide to donate embryos for research only after they have decided not to continue storing their embryos. Making separate decisions about no longer using embryos and donating them for research guards against pressure placed on couples to donate embryos. When embryos are created, couples often stipulate what should be done with their frozen embryos in the event of future contingencies, such as death, divorce, or no contact with the clinic. These directives usually involve donating the embryos to another couple, donating them for research, or discarding them. If no death or divorce occurs, the couple makes a separate decision about what should be done with the unused embryos when their fertility needs are met or they end their reproductive efforts with these embryos. At this point, the investigator has the opportunity to discuss more thoroughly the option of donating embryos for research.

Using only frozen embryos for research ensures that time passes between the creation of embryos for conception and their donation for research. Still, it is reasonable to expect questions eventually to arise about the donation of fresh but supernumerary embryos.[16] Donation of fresh embryos raises the possibility that a physician might induce a patient to allow insemination of extra eggs so that they may be donated for research. Moreover, this increases the chance that decisions will be made quickly and later regretted by couples. Without evidence that fresh embryos are significantly preferable to frozen embryos for ES cell use, it is appropriate to use only spare embryos that have been frozen. The number of embryos created and frozen should be determined by the clinical needs of the infertile couple.

In some situations, couples with stored embryos cannot be contacted despite efforts on the part of the clinic. The Ethics Committee has previously concluded that programs may consider embryos abandoned if clinics have taken diligent steps to contact the couple, no written instructions exist, and more than 5 years have elapsed without contact with the couple.[17] Abandoned embryos may be discarded, but they should not be used for research or donated to another couple without prior consent. In some cases, however, couples may have given consent to use spare embryos for research but were not informed of the possibility of ES cell research. The singular features of ES cell research make it advisable not to use such embryos for ES cell research unless couples have given specific advance consent for this purpose, in case they cannot later be reached for a decision. Advance permission to use abandoned embryos for research may thus prevail for ES cell studies if the couple has been informed of the possibility of ES cell research.

Who Should Secure Consent

Several advisory bodies have recommended that a person other than the fertility specialist secure consent to donate embryos.[2, 13] The rationale is that this will ensure that the couple's reproductive needs are foremost and avoid conflicts of interest when the fertility specialist is also the investigator. In some circumstances, however, this guideline may be difficult to follow. It is possible, for example, that the fertility specialist, who knows the couple and is trusted by them may be better able to have a frank discussion with the couple about donation for research and may secure more informed consent.

Moreover, using a separate person to secure consent may be difficult if the physician is part of the research team. The possibility of undue influence by the physician will be lessened if the request for a donation is made after the couple decides to dispose of their embryos. Still, the fact that the physician is also a researcher is relevant information and should be conveyed to the couple along with a statement about financial incentives, if any, the physician has in the research, The rule that the number of embryos created and frozen must be determined by the clinical needs of the couple and not by research goals is especially pertinent when the physician is both the fertility specialist and investigator.

SUMMARY

The Ethic Committee believes it is ethically acceptable to derive and use ES cells in research to develop cell replacement therapies and to further other medical uses. This research should take place only within guidelines in peace for embryo research in general and only under conditions that protect the free and informed consent of couples. At a minimum, guidelines for informed consent include the following about what should be conveyed to couples, when, and by whom.

1. The consent process should inform donors of the nature of ES cell derivation; the specific research project, if known; source of funding; potential commercial value; and anticipated clinical implications. Policies on confidentiality and maintenance of the donors' privacy should be developed by the clinic and presented as part of the consent process.
2. The final decisions on the donation of embryos to ES cell or other research must occur after the couple's infertility needs are met or the couple discontinues therapy, except in rare cases where the couple is not available and has given explicit written directions in advance for use of their embryos in ES cell research.
3. Whenever possible, someone other than the treating infertility specialist should make requests for embryos for research purposes. Couples should be informed that refusal to participate will not affect medical

care and that embryos used for research will not be transferred to a woman's uterus for possible pregnancy. They should be informed of financial incentives, if any, that the physician has in the research.
4. Embryos should not be bought or sold with a monetary exchange. Reasonable fees may be charged for laboratory processing or for handling, storage, or transport of embryos.

NOTES

1. Thomson JA, Itskovitz-Eldor J, Shapiro SS, Waknitz, MA, Swiergiel JJ, Marshill VS, et al. Embryonic stem cell lines derived from human blastocysts. Science 1998;282:1145–7.

2. American Association for the Advancement of Science and Institute for Civil Society. Stem cell, research and applications; monitoring the frontiers of biomedical research. Washington, DC: American Association for the Advancement of Science 1999:3.

3. National Institutes of Health. Office of the Director. Stem cells: a primer. May 2000. Available at http://www.nih.gov/news/stemcell/primer.htm. Accessed on November 2, 2000.

4. The White House. Office of the Press Secretary. Radio address by the President to the nation. Bush Ranch, Crawford, Texas, August 11, 2001. Available at http://www.whitehousegov/news/releases/2000. Accessed on February 5, 2002.

5. Ethics Committee of the American Fertility Society. Ethical considerations of the new reproductive technologies. Fertil Steril 1986;4(1 Suppl):1S.

6. Ethics Committee of the American Fertility Society. Ethical considerations of the new reproductive technologies. Fertil Steril 1990;53(2 Suppl):1S.

7. Ethics Committee of the American Fertility Society. Ethical considerations of assisted reproductive technologies. Fertil Steril 1994;62(1Suppl):1S.

8. Ethics Committee of the American Society Reproductive Medicine. Informed consent and the use of gametes and embryos for research, Fertil Steril 1997; 68:780–1.

9. ESHRE Task Force on Ethics and Law. 1. The moral status of the pre-implantation embryo. Hum Reprod 2001;16:1046–8.

10. ESHRE Task Force on Ethics and Law. IV. Stem cells. Hum Reprod 2002; 17:1409–10.

11. United Kingdom Department of Health. Government response to the recommendations made in the Chief Medical Officer's Expert Group report, "Stem Cell Research. Medical Progress with Responsibility." August 2000.

12. Australian Academy of Science. On human cloning: a position statement. Canberra: Australian Academy of Science, February 4, 1999.

13. National Bioethics Advisory Commission. Ethical issues in human cell research: report and recommendations of the National Bioethics Advisory Commission. Rockville, MD: National Bioethics Advisory Commission, 1999.

14. National Institutes of Health. Draft National Institutes of Health guidelines for research involving human pluripotent stem cells. Fed Regist 1999;64;67576–9.

15. Canadian Institutes of Health Research. Human stem cell research: opportunities for health and ethical perspectives: a discussion paper. Ottawa: Canadian Institutes of Health Research, 2001.

16. National Institutes of Health guidelines for research using human pluripotent stem cells. Fed Regist 2000;65:6995.

17. Ethics Committee of the American Society for Reproductive Medicine. Disposition of abandoned embryos. Fertil Steril 1997:67(1 Suppl):1S.

Index

AAMC. *See* Association of American
Medical Colleges
academia and industry, 63–66, 71–72,
114; factors, 66–71
acquired immunodeficiency virus
(AIDS). *See* human
immunodeficiency virus
adolescents: and sexual health care,
87–92, 93–98; sexual health care
statistics, 87–89, 92–95; advance
directives, 119, *123–24*, 125, 128
Afghanistan, 48
Africa, 27–31, 37–39, 40
age, 5–6, 21n4; selling organs and, *101*,
102; tube feeding and, *122–23*,
124–25, 128. *See also* tube feeding
AIDS. *See* human immunodeficiency
virus
allotransplantation. *See* transplants.
Al Qaeda, 48
Alzheimer's disease, 117, 119, 125, 128,
139; and race, 37, 39–40
AMA. *See* American Medical
Association
American Academy of Family
Physicians, 89
American Academy of Pediatrics, 89
American College of Obstetricians and
Gynecologists, 89

American Medical Association (AMA),
88–89; National Coalition on
Adolescent Health, 89; National
Council on Scientific Affairs, 89
American Society for Reproductive
Medicine (ASRM), 141, 143, 144
Amnesty International, 112
anthrax, 46, 55
antibiotics, 136
Argentina, 112, 113
Asia, 28–29, 31, 37, 39
ASRM. *See* American Society for
Reproductive Medicine
Association of American Medical
Colleges (AAMC), 63, 66, 69, 71
Association of American Universities,
63, 66
Aurora Biosciences, 67

baboons, medical use, 134
Bangladesh, 115
Bill and Melinda Gates Foundation, 67
bioterrorism, 45–48, 50. *See also* Model
State Emergency Health Powers Act
birth control. *See* adolescents
bovine spongiform encephalopathy, 135
Brazil, 112, 113, 116
British National Health Service, 6, 7
Brown, Christopher C., 114

148   *Index*

bubonic plague, 46, 48, 51
Bush, George W., 139
Business-Higher Education Forum, 63

cancer, 139
cats, medical use, 135
CDC. *See* Centers for Disease Control
and Prevention
Center for Law and the Public's Health,
45–46, 51
Center for the Study of Society and
Medicine, 114
Centers for Disease Control and
Prevention (CDC), 45, 46, 50, 133–35
Central America, 28
Central Intelligence Agency (CIA), 47
chimpanzees, and HIV, 135–36
China, 29, 112
CIA. *See* Central Intelligence Agency
Clinton, William J., 139
clinical trials. *See* research
Cohen, Lawrence, 112, 115–16
Columbia University, 114
Commission on Macroeconomics and
Health, 30
contraceptives. *See* adolescents
Costa Rica, 9
Creutzfeldt-Jakob disease, 136
Crohn's disease, 39
Cuba, 9, 112
Current Anthropology, 113

Dark Winter, 48, 51
death, 10, 118, 129, 143
dementia. *See* tube feeding
Democratic Republic of the Congo, 30
diabetes, 37, 139
disability, 4–7, 21nn1–2
disease, 4, 6, 21n1, 46–47, 80, 139;
cross-species, 47, 133–36; rare, 75,
77–78, 80. *See also* bovine
spongiform encephalopathy; human
immunodeficiency virus; porcine
endogenous retrovirus; race; sexually
transmitted diseases

divorce. *See* marital status
DNR order. *See* advance directives; do-
not-resuscitate order
do-not-resuscitate order, 125, 128–29,
130. *See also* advance directives
Draper Laboratory, 67

eBay, 114
education, 10–11, *101*, 102
elderly. *See* age
embryonic stem (ES) cells, 139–45
embryos: donor consent, 139, 141–45;
fresh, 143; frozen, 143–44; research,
140–45; sale of, 141, 145; societal
status, 140–41; sources, 139–40,
142–43
endogenous retroviruses. *See* porcine
endogenous retrovirus
ES cells. *See* embryonic stem (ES) cells
Estonia, 28
ethics, 80, 100–101, 111–16, 140–45;
and health care fairness, 1–2, 6,
12–20, 22n6. *See also* Rawls's theory
of justice
ethnicity. *See* race
Europe, 28, 37, 112

family planning services. *See*
adolescents
FDA. *See* U.S. Food and Drug
Administration
Food and Drug Administration. *See* U.S.
Food and Drug Administration

gender, 105, 119; in research, 90; selling
organs and, *101*, 102–3; tube feeding
and, *122–23*, 124
Georgetown University, 45–46
GFATM. *See* Global Fund to Fight
AIDS, Tuberculosis and Malaria
Global Alliance for TB Drug
Development, 67
Global Fund to Fight AIDS,
Tuberculosis and Malaria (GFATM),
29–31

Great Britain. *See* British National
   Health Service

HAART. *See* highly active antiretroviral
   therapy
Harlan, John Marshall, 55
Harvard Medical School, 71
health: inequalities, 7–12; international,
   9, 11–12, 27–31, 37–41;law, 48–50;
   normal functioning, 3–7; social
   determinants, 2, 7–12. *See also* age;
   income; Model State Emergency
   Health Powers Act; race; transplants
health care: decision-making, 13, 15–20,
   22n7; distribution, 1–2, 6, 12–20,
   22n6; economics, 5, 14, 18, 21n3;
   function, 1–2, 22n5; moral
   importance, 1, 3–7; social obligation,
   5–6; types, 5–6, 19–20; universal,
   5–6, 7, 10, 12. *See also* adolescents;
   age; bioterrorism; income; race;
   Rawls's theory of justice; tube
   feeding
Health Information Portability and
   Accountability Act of 1995, 65
hepatitis, 136
Hereditary Disease Foundation, 67
herpes, 136
highly active antiretroviral therapy
   (HAART), 27–28, 30
HIV. *See* human immunodeficiency
   virus
human immunodeficiency virus (HIV),
   27–31, 39, 135–36
Huntington Study Group, 67

income, 2, 8–11, 36–37. *See also*
   transplants
India, 9, 29, 99–102, 104–6, 112,
   115–16; statistics, 99, 101, 102–4
industry. *See* academia
influenza, 46–47
insurance, 5–6, 7, 10, 12, 19–20
International AIDS Conference, 27, 31
in vitro fertilization (IVF), 140, 142–43

Iraq, 9
Israel, 112
IVF. *See* in vitro fertilization

Jacobson v. Massachusetts (1905), 55
Japan, 39–40
Johns Hopkins University, 45–46, 67
justice. *See* ethics; Rawls's theory of
   justice

Kamm, Oliver, 15, 21n4

The Lancet, 116
Latvia, 28
Lederberg, Joshua, 133
liberties, civil, 7–8, 55–58
life expectancy, 8–9
Lincoln Laboratory, 67
living will. *See* advance directives
Loyola University of Chicago, 115

"mad cow disease." *See* bovine
   spongiform encephalopathy
Maine Supreme Court, 56
marital status, and health issues, 106,
   143; tube feeding and, 117, 119–20,
   122, 124, 124–25
marriage. *See* marital status
Marshall, Mac, 113
Marshall, Patricia, 115
Massachusetts Institute of Technology, 67
Massachusetts Supreme Judicial Court,
   55–56
MDS. *See* National Repository Resident
   Assessment Instrument Minimum
   Data Set
measles, 46
Medicaid, 117–19, *123–24*, 125, 128
Medicare, 117, 119
mice, medical use, 135
microbes, resistance to drugs, 136
Middle East, 112
Model State Emergency Health Powers
   Act (MSEHPA), 45–46, *51–52*,
   53–58

About the Contributors

1. Norman Daniels is a Professor of Ethics and Population Health at the Harvard University School of Public Health.
2. Kevin M. De Cock is with the Centers for Disease Control in Kenya, Nairobi.
3. Robert S. Janssen is with the National Center for HIV, STD, & TB Prevention at the Centers for Disease Control in Atlanta, GA.
4. Esteban González Burchard is at the Lung Biology Center, the University of California, San Francisco, San Francisco, CA.
5. Elad Ziv is in the Division of General Medicine at the San Francisco General Hospital
6. Natasha Coyle is at the Lung Biology Center at the San Francisco General Hospital.
7. Scarlet Lin Gomez is in the Division of Epidemiology, Department of Health Research and Policy at Stanford University School of Medicine
8. Hua Tang is in the Department of Statistics at Stanford University School of Medicine.
9. Andrew J. Karter is at the Department of Epidemiology and Health Services Research, Division of Research, Kaiser Permanente in Oakland, CA.
10. Joanna L. Mountain is in the Department of Anthropological Sciences at Stanford University School of Medicine.
11. Eliseo J. Pérez-Stable is in the Division of General Medicine at the San Francisco General Hospital.
12. Dean Sheppard is in the Department of Medicine at the San Francisco General Hospital.

13. Lawrence O. Gostin is at the Center for Law and the Public's Health at Georgetown University, Washington, D.C.
14. Neil Risch is in the Department of Genetics at Stanford University School of Medicine.
15. Jason W. Sapsin is at the Center for Law and The Public's Health at Georgetown University and the Johns Hopkins University.
16. Stephen P. Teret is at the Center for Law and The Public's Health at Georgetown University and the Johns Hopkins University.
17. Scott Burris is at the Center for Law and The Public's Health at Georgetown University and the Johns Hopkins University.
18. Julie Samia Mair is at the Center for Law and The Public's Health at Georgetown University and the Johns Hopkins University.
19. James G. Hodge, Jr. is at the Center for Law and The Public's Health at Georgetown University and the Johns Hopkins University.
20. Jon S. Vernick is at the Center for Law and The Public's Health at Georgetown University and the Johns Hopkins University.
21. Hamilton Moses III is the Senior Advisor at the Boston Consulting Group in Bethesda, MD.
22. Eugene Braunwald is at Partners HealthCare System, Boston, MA.
23. Joseph B. Martin is at Harvard Medical School, Boston, MA.
24. Samuel O. Thier is at Partners HealthCare System, Boston, MA.
25. Scott D. Halpern is at the Center for Clinical Epidemiology and Biostatistics and the Center for Bioethics at the University of Pennsylvania School of Medicine, Philadelphia, PA.
26. Jason H. T. Karlawish is that the Center for Bioethics at the University of Pennsylvania School of Medicine, Philadelphia, PA.
27. Jesse A. Berlin is at the Center for Clinical Epidemiology and Biostatistics at the University of Pennsylvania School of Medicine, Philadelphia, PA.
28. Diane M. Reddy is in the Department of Psychology at the University of Wisconsin-Milwaukee, Milwaukee, WI.
29. Raymond Fleming is at the Department of Psychology, University of Wisconsin–Milwaukee, Milwaukee, WI.
30. Carolyne Swain is at Midwestern Professional Research and Educational Services, Inc. Milwaukee, WI.
31. Madhav Goyal is in the Department of Internal Medicine, Geisinger Health System, State College, PA.
32. Ravindra L. Mehta is at the Department of Nephrology, University of California, San Diego, School of Medicine.
33. Lawrence J. Schneiderman is at the Departments of Family and Preventive Medicine and Medicine, University of California, San Diego, School of Medicine

34. Ashwini R. Sehgal is at the Division of Nephrology and Center for Health Care Research and Policy, Case Western Reserve University, Cleveland, OH.
35. Peter Monaghan frequently writes for the *Chronicle of Higher Education*.
36. Susan L. Mitchell is at the Hebrew Rehabilitation Center for the Aged, Boston, MA.
37. Joan M. Teno is at the Center for Gerontology and Health Care Research, Department of Community Health, Brown Medical School, Providence, RI.
38. Jason Roy is at the Center for Gerontology and Health Care Research, Department of Community Health, Brown Medical School, Providence, RI.
39. Glen Kabumoto is at the Center for Gerontology and Health Care Research, Department of Community Health, Brown Medical School, Providence, RI.
40. Vincent Mor is at the Center for Gerontology and Health Care Research, Department of Community Health, Brown Medical School, Providence, RI.
41. Robin A. Weiss is at the Wohl Virion Center, Windeyer Institute of Medical Sciences, University College, London, UK.